BEYOND IMPLEMENTATION:

A Prescription for Lasting
EMR ADOPTION

Heather A. Haugen, PhD
Jeffrey R. Woodside, MD

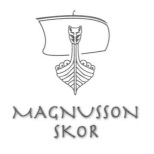

MAGNUSSON
SKOR

Denver
www.magnussonskor.com

Published by

MAGNUSSON
SKOR

Magnusson Skor Publishing
4600 S. Ulster Street Suite 1300
Denver, CO 80237
www.magnussonskor.com

To purchase Magnusson Skor products, visit our website at
www.magnussonskor.com. Discounts on bulk quantities are available
to corporations, professional associations, and other organizations.
For details and discounts, please contact us.

Library of Congress Cataloging-in-Publication Data

Haugen, Heather A., 1973-
Woodside, Jeffrey R., 1942-

  Beyond Implementation: A Prescription for Lasting EMR Adoption.
  p. cm.
  Includes biographical references.
  ISBN 978-0-9842051-0-3
  1. EMR adoption 2. Healthcare 3. Health Information Technology I. Title

First Edition

*This book is dedicated to our colleagues
at The Breakaway Group*

C O N T E N T S

Despite the significant benefits of electronic medical records, organizations continue to struggle with successful technology adoption. Beyond Implementation examines the primary reason for poor and failed EMR adoption, explores real-world results from large healthcare organizations, and reveals a new approach for successful adoption and lasting value.

The authors, Dr. Heather Haugen and Dr. Jeffrey Woodside, have witnessed the outcomes of poor adoption and are committed to helping organizations successfully adopt an EMR system. Through actual case studies and research, the book investigates the barriers that keep physicians from making EMR part of their routines. The key premise: a myopic focus on go-live implementation impedes the adoption and long-term sustainment of EMR.

Implementation vs. Adoption

"Implementation happens when the application is installed and live; an important milestone from a technology perspective, but only a small step toward adoption. Adoption is the continuous process of keeping users informed and engaged, providing innovative ways for them to become proficient in new tasks quickly, measuring changes in critical outcomes, and striving to sustain that level of performance long-term. Adoption is not a snapshot at a single point in time; it is a motion picture."

Research-Based Approach

"By interviewing physician leaders, Chief Medical Information Officers and Chief Medical Officers at organizations representing over 3,200 physicians and 350 ambulatory sites, we studied the gap between perceived adoption and actual use of an EMR and as a result, we gained a better understanding of the common barriers to EMR adoption and the strategies for overcoming them."

The Potential of EMR

"We are living in an era that is a critical turning point in Health Information Technology. We have the technology, legislation, funding, resources and sense of urgency to make a giant leap in how we apply technology to healthcare...For those willing to seize the opportunity, now is the time to break away."

Preventing "Go-Live Myopia"

"When decision-makers focus on just one event, a successful go-live, it is very easy to forego the processes that ensure adoption. Too many organizational leaders still believe that once the application goes live, users will embrace it. However, it becomes strikingly obvious after a go-live when the key elements of adoption have been left out. Many organizations have implemented an EMR, but very few have successfully adopted the EMR."

How Leaders Create a "Tone at the Top"

"Leaders currently in charge of EMR adoption need to develop a ferocious understanding of what they are going to stop doing, and then maintain the courage to follow through on their decisions. Because it demonstrates active commitment to end users who are affected by the new workflows, this may be the single greatest action toward successful adoption of an EMR."

A Simulation-Based Approach

"...simulators literally change how healthcare providers learn new technology. First, they are designed separately for each role that will use the application...Individuals do not have to learn to use every function in an application, but they do have to learn all functions related to their specific role. It is a mistake to teach every function of the entire application..."

Performance Metrics and Adoption

"The commitment to identify even just a few key metrics will provide enormous value to the organization. First, it will be very handy in proving meaningful use. Second, it can be used as a dashboard for measuring the performance of the EMR for the life of the application. Most importantly, it will drive continual improvement in the specific areas of value to the organization."

The UT Medical Group Story

"...the acquisition, implementation and adoption of any new technology is a journey of many steps. We know that all new staff will learn how to use our EMR consistently and according to uniform policies. The time it will take for them to get up to speed is much shorter, allowing them to spend more time treating patients and less time on the computer. I am thrilled to say that we have truly improved our organization and its operation to the ultimate benefit of our patients."

Planning for Sustainment

"Effective sustainability plans require resources, time and money. Keep in mind that adoption is never static; it is either improving or degrading in the organization...Leadership must plan for the investment and fund it if their ultimate goal is improved performance. Most organizations only achieve modest adoption after a go-live event, and it takes relentless focus to achieve the levels of adoption needed to improve quality of care, patient safety and financial outcomes."

Collaborating on this book has been one of life's greatest adventures and challenges. We would like to recognize the many contributions by our colleagues, mentors and families. We are so thankful for the expertise, counsel and unwavering support we have received. It is our greatest hope that this book makes a difference in the lives of clinicians - the real heroes of healthcare.

This book would not have been possible without our editor, Inbal Vuletich. Inbal was literally the glue that held this effort together. Editor, writer, counselor and project manager were just a few of the roles she filled. Her commitment to this project was truly a gift.

Charles Fred inspired this effort. He believed in the research and the book before we did. As one of our toughest critics, his feedback was always on target and it made us better. Thanks for the sizzle, Mr. Fred!

Early in this project, we recognized the importance of using real-life examples from healthcare to demonstrate our point of view. Steve Burkett, the CEO of UT Medical Group, was generous enough to share the real challenges of EMR adoption from his perspective. The story of UTMG demonstrates not only the challenges, but also the opportunities for the future of EMR adoption. Steve and his team are true pioneers.

Personal Acknowledgements

Heather:

I am so grateful for the support of my family. I am lucky to have a husband who appreciates my passion for this work and always encourages me through the tough spots. He is also an amazing dad which brings me the peace of mind that only a working mom can appreciate. My parents have been two of the most important role models in my life and continue to be my greatest resources.

Jeff:

I want to thank my lovely wife and best friend for her support during the writing of this book and for her abiding good humor regarding the time I spent secluded in my office. Donna, I promise we will be spending more time pursuing the enjoyable activities of our alleged retirement! I am grateful to Charles for inviting me to join The Breakaway Group. My colleagues have become my friends and it is a joy to be part of this company that truly lives our promise to always leave more than we take - not only with our clients, but also with our fellow team members and our communities.

BEYOND IMPLEMENTATION:

A Prescription for Lasting
EMR ADOPTION

INTRODUCTION

The POLYCOM beeps its standard two-syllable signoff as the conference call ends; the silence is calming after the discussion generated by the recap of a three-year journey to electronic medical record (EMR) adoption. It's 6:30 pm on a Monday and we just finished a research call with a physician leader representing a practice group. The call was important as it concluded nearly 14 months of investigation to find new and innovative methods for EMR adoption within physician practices – and to identify the barriers that keep physicians from making the technology part of their daily routine. The call we just completed reinforced earlier messages we heard: "true adoption of an EMR by physician-providers will remain elusive without a collective strategy to remove identifiable, yet significant barriers." Physicians across myriad practices and specialties recite common barriers with near synchronicity as they grapple with changes in workflow, interoperability with other applications and ultimately, the use of their time.

> "We believe our study has uncovered a leading cause of poor or failed physician adoption of EMRs: the early and persistent focus, by vendors and clinical leadership, on implementation as the indicator of success."

We believe our study has uncovered a leading cause of poor or failed physician adoption of EMRs: the early and persistent focus, by vendors and clinical leadership, on implementation as the indicator of success.

A singular effort by the vendor community and the provider leadership to ensure that the application is operational has created an atmosphere where go-live becomes the end game and all associated budget and activities are directed toward that goal. This mental model will forever produce applications that are only partially utilized, with clinician resistance and shortfalls of expected financial returns. This level of thinking assumes there is a defined event whereby the application is adopted and used.

Our research tells a different story. The drive toward implementation creates expectations and false assumptions that blind decision-makers to the end user's real needs and long-term sustainment required for the continual flux in staffing and workflow. Leaders rejoicing at go-live also fail to see the importance of longer term budgeting, ongoing measures of effectiveness, a multi-stakeholder governance structure and cultural adjustments needed for true adoption. The chasm between a one-time implementation approach versus the ongoing leadership of adoption is often vast. Our aim is to unfold a new approach toward managing and leading successful adoption.

Let's begin by changing our primary target from implementation to adoption. Implementation happens when the application is installed and live; an important milestone from a technology perspective, but only a small step toward adoption. Adoption is the continuous process of keeping users informed and engaged, providing innovative ways for them

"Let's begin by changing our primary target from implementation to adoption."

3

to become proficient in new tasks quickly, measuring changes in critical outcomes, and striving to sustain that level of performance long-term. Adoption is not a snapshot at a single point in time; it is a motion picture.

There is good news. The American Recovery and Reinvestment Act of 2009 (ARRA) funding provides both the financial incentive and the sense of urgency needed to transform how we utilize EMRs. It is more important than ever for physicians and practice managers to address the gap between merely implementing and fully adopting a new EMR.

This book introduces a method for adopting an EMR and for creating a foundation for continuous improvement of quality, safety and efficiency in an organization. Our research results provide a framework that makes it easy for executives and physician leaders to initiate a dialogue around lasting EMR adoption.

Yours in Good Health,

Heather and Jeff

CHAPTER ONE

A Journey To EMR Adoption

Chapter Preview: • The UT Medical Group Story
• Research Conclusions

" *There is no more delicate matter to take in hand, nor more dangerous to conduct, nor more doubtful in its success, than to set up as a leader in the introduction of changes. For he who innovates will have for enemies all those who are well off under the existing order of things, and only lukewarm supporters in those who might be better off under the new.*"

~ Niccolo Machiavelli 1532

The UT Medical Group Story

Asmidgeon east of downtown Memphis, sandwiched between Union and Popular avenues, is a sober administrative building wearing the address *66 North Pauline Street*. The structure provides a command center for UT Medical Group, Inc. (UTMG), the faculty group practice of the University of Tennessee College of Medicine. To an outsider, the dowdy nature of the building and its obscure location might seem incongruent with the type of tenant operating inside, especially when one considers that the group's 375 physicians are actively involved in teaching and research for advanced treatment and provision of most organ transplants in the Mid-South. To the benefit of Mid-South residents who require specialized care and state-of-the-art clinical services, the UTMG staff has invested in the development of successful programs such as the neonatal and high-risk birth centers, trauma and burn units at The Regional Medical Center, the liver, kidney and pancreas transplant programs at Methodist University Hospital and the heart center at Le Bonheur Children's Medical Center. To say the least, investing in an ostentatious administrative building is not big on their list of priorities. Investing in an application that could potentially save lives and improve care – now, that is something they will quickly consider.

Enter the promise of the EMR and all of its trimmings. Given UTMG's history as teachers, researchers and early adopters of technology, they became the ideal target for the early use of nascent EMR technologies. In fact, the combination of the accomplishments of the group, the experience of the leaders and the recent push to adopt new Health Information Technology (HIT) formed the perfect storm. Led by veteran and highly respected president and CEO, Steven Burkett, the group entered the tempest with confidence, believing they could effectively implement an enterprise application and quickly reap the clinical benefits. Into the storm they went.

To quote the late Paul Harvey, "Now here is the rest of the story," as told by Steven Burkett. This account is the best representation of an EMR case study that we have discovered over our 14-month research adventure. The venerable Burkett – always the teacher – graciously agreed to share his personal perspective regarding the complexities of UTMG's EMR adoption and subsequent re-implementation. Steven gives an authentic and forthright account of UTMG's experience from the initial frustration and resistance to the physicians embracing and adopting the new EMR.

◆

This is the story of UTMG's journey from unsuccessful implementation to successful EMR adoption – from the agony of defeat to the thrill of victory! I have been fortunate to serve as CEO of UT Medical Group for some 25 years. Twenty-five years ago, our hospitals and clinics all utilized paper charting and coding. The process of charge capture was onerous, to say the least. We had doctors writing hurried, illegible notes, nurses trying to decipher scribbled orders, and administrative staff struggling to assign correct coding for services and levels of care.

By the late 1990's, many of our physicians and other clinicians from different departments came to me and other members of the management team, each believing that they had found the best electronic method or solution for patient information tracking and charge capture. However, there was no practical way, certainly no standard means, to create interfaces from each of these individual solutions with our IDX practice management system. We needed a solution that would allow for easy acquisition of patient demographic, diagnostic and procedural data from a variety of geographic locations, while allowing for easy, safe interface directly with the practice management system. The automated charge capture process held the promise of improved efficiency, improved process quality and cost savings. We began to consider a radical change in our methods – and this led us to the acquisition of an EMR.

At the time, Allscripts was one of the few EMR vendors with academic medical practice experience and an established relationship with IDX. We quickly realized the value of working with Allscripts and IDX to capitalize on their existing business relationship, thus avoiding costly custom interfaces. It was of paramount importance to maintain the integrity of the transactions and to keep labor costs low as we went through this transition. I wanted the opportunity to show the entire organization what the future of medical records could do for us by providing the charge module within a familiar system.

It has long been my belief that patient data should be easily accessible to our physicians from any location at any time and that making the information available in a cost-effective way would be in the best interest of our patients and our physicians, giving our organization a competitive advantage. For our academic physicians, practice is but one aspect of their professional activities; the patient information in the electronic system is vital because they practice in many venues and on changing schedules. Physicians who work in the same practice locale every day are more likely to have access to paper records and to recall details about their patients. Our geographic dispersion and changing schedules suggested to me that our physicians would welcome readily available clinical information at their fingertips, regardless of their location. While generally speaking this is true, I didn't appreciate the degree to which the adoption of such technology would require changing personal habits and workflow, becoming major barriers to this transition.

> "I didn't appreciate the degree to which the adoption of such technology would require changing personal habits and workflow, thus becoming major barriers to this transition."

There was broad participation by medical staff, revenue cycle personnel and management in the selection process of the EMR vendor, and the Board approved the capital expenditure. We all wanted to make improvements using appropriate technology that would reduce labor costs and minimize human data entry error while supporting clinical activity and improved claims submission. Our financial analysis included cost savings from elimination of paper records, reduction of personnel in medical records, and elimination of human handling of items such as radiology reports. When those savings were projected across our hospitals, hospital-based clinics and private clinics, the value proposition of an EMR became compelling. A vendor was selected and we were ready to move ahead.

We developed an implementation plan which called for Information Technology (IT) to manage the project, including end user training and the technical aspects of hardware, software and implementation. We identified a part-time Chief Medical Information Officer (CMIO) with a background in health informatics to serve as a physician leader and at least one physician in each department to go through a train-the-trainer program. These people were responsible for leading their departments through the education on the software. The training firm retained was one recommended by our vendor. At the time, I thought that our leadership and the appeal of the new system would drive physician adoption of the new system; sadly, I was wrong. While there was certainly excitement and

11

enthusiasm about the potential of the new system, it could not overcome the habit and culture change required for not only adoption but also effective implementation of the new technology. Our failure to adequately address changing workflows, the handling of information and the need to change individual work habits led to poor adoption and underutilization. Lack of standardization was also a significant contributor to our difficulties. I hadn't appreciated the degree to which our different clinics and locations had very different workflows and that proceeding without first standardizing these workflows presented very serious obstacles.

> "I thought that our leadership and the appeal of the new system would drive physician adoption of the new system; sadly, I was wrong. "

In addition, we underestimated the resources and the discipline required for UTMG to fully adopt, particularly in the context of our distributed geography. As long as IT personnel were on site to support users, they were content to use the system, because when they got stuck, there was someone standing by to help. However, this was an unrealistic environment; we couldn't afford to continue to have IT support staff on site at all times. In spite of good relationships between the clinic staff and IT, end user habits still did not change and adoption by the end user was not, in reality, proceeding. I have always heard that it is easier to build a hospital than to operate one; similarly, our new technology was easy to install but difficult to adopt.

I was pleasantly surprised at how rapidly many house staff and fellows adopted the EMR. In one department, the house staff's enthusiasm to implement the system became the real driving force. This in turn elevated the interest of many of the faculty. We also had groups in the organization that used the EMR and used it well. They were our earliest adopters. Pediatric cardiology was first to be paperless in clinics, quickly expanding their use for teaching conferences and becoming champions for the EMR.

We had a good technical staff, good technology and an interested medical staff. However, our communications were inconsistent and sometimes inaccurate. We lacked a well-defined, well-functioning problem-solving group and escalation process, not to mention a standardized communication program. We needed a new strategy for our physician leadership to communicate the changes throughout the whole organization, and to stay involved throughout the change process. We had embarked on not only the implementation and adoption of an EMR, but a culture change as well.

Interestingly enough, physician leaders were not expressing concerns during implementation, certainly not on a widespread basis, nor to the degree anticipated. As it turned out, we were not implementing the system consistently across the various disciplines and locations. Each area was customizing as they felt was needed, so it appeared things were working just fine. With constant IT support, we had what initially appeared to be a successful adoption process. But because we lacked standardization, we had minimized the value of the EMR. Physicians and clinic staff had not embraced change; they had simply molded the system to fit around their existing paper-based workflows.

"Physicians and clinic staff had not embraced change; they had simply molded the system to fit around their existing paper-based workflows."

In addition, few seemed to understand the value of the medical record information as data. Many physicians, nurses and clinical staff saw the EMR as simply a "faster paper record" rather than as a new resource for caring for our patients. Many did not appreciate the overall potential cost savings to UTMG. In order to understand the value proposition, we had to look at our entire process of delivering care, not just the portion of the process involving the physician/patient interaction. When we looked at the continuum of events, consistently recording demographic and patient information was where we initially gained the greatest efficiencies and therefore cost savings (reduced labor cost and human error). In some areas, improved clinical documentation led to increased revenue. Understanding and communicating the value proposition to the medical staff is a critical element for success. It was a weakness in our initial implementation effort.

As the implementation progressed, the lack of standardization and structure began to take its toll. The IT team was

14

frustrated because leadership failed to impose the necessary rules for use of the system. End users weren't really adopting the system and it became more of an "IT Project" rather than a technology used to care for our patients which was supported by IT. Our Chief Information Officer (CIO) and project manager departed for other opportunities, so we put the implementation on hold. During the period of recruiting a new CIO, the project went into maintenance mode.

"it is embarrassing to admit, but the lack of negative feedback about the implementation was actually a sign of difficulty."

In retrospect, it is embarrassing to admit, but the lack of negative feedback about the implementation was actually a sign of difficulty. The positive feedback received had more to do with good reviews of IT staff than use of the system. This should have been a signal that people were not becoming self-sufficient in the use of the new system, yet I was encouraged and felt that the implementation was going well. The value of negative feedback cannot be overstated; it can identify the pain points and provide the opportunity to address issues. While the year-long hiatus in implementation was very disappointing, it provided me and the organization the opportunity to thoroughly assess the position we were in, the problems we experienced and the time to carefully plan our next steps. It was clear that I needed to become more familiar with the EMR so that I could address potential issues before they derailed adoption. Going forward, I committed to being more involved, better informed and better prepared.

To Be Continued...

UTMG's experience is not unique. Our research suggests that many organizations are experiencing these same challenges: lack of project governance, user resistance, lack of established and enforced policies and procedures, silos of adoption, silos of communication and lack of metrics to track outcomes. Adoption does not have to be painful, but it does require the discipline to follow a proven methodology.

Our research with large physician practice groups has been an extremely valuable effort. We targeted those who had implemented or were in the process of implementing an EMR. By interviewing physician leaders, Chief Medical Information Officers and Chief Medical Officers at organizations representing over 3200 physicians and 350 ambulatory sites, we studied the gap between perceived adoption and actual use of an EMR and as a result, we gained a better understanding of the common barriers to EMR adoption and the strategies for overcoming them.

> "Adoption does not have to be painful, but it does require the discipline to follow a proven methodology."

In addition to this research project, our client experiences contributed to the evolution of our research conclusions. Our experience spans many applications, including Radiology Information Systems, Electronic Medical Records and Practice Management Solutions, and every type of project, from new installations to upgrades and even painful re-implementations. We also have a bias for metrics when it comes to working with clients, so we developed a rigorous process for measuring outcomes. Two key indicators of adoption are the knowledge and confidence of end users; we measure both at baseline, after go-live and on a regular basis. The metrics provide an objective assessment of adoption.

The culmination of these efforts provided us with a clearer understanding of the critical components and processes necessary to overcome the barriers to adoption and led to the development of a robust methodology to produce lasting adoption.

Research Conclusions

1. Implementation and adoption are not synonymous, but almost universally treated as the same effort.
2. Very few organizations track end-user adoption in terms of clinical and financial outcomes.
3. Physician adoption is highly dependent on the degree of engaged leadership. Physician leaders need to be involved early in the process and be empowered to make decisions that impact the use of the application.
4. Traditional training methods, like classroom training, don't produce proficient users. Inadequate education of end users is a significant contributor to poor EMR adoption and ultimately poor business outcomes.
5. Successful organizations develop 3-5 year plans for sustaining adoption long past the implementation.

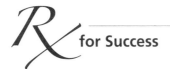

for Success

- Put a strategy in play for adoption not just implementation.
- Learn from other healthcare organizations going through an EMR adoption. Visit other organizations that have been successful in their journey!
- Utilize research findings to overcome common barriers to EMR adoption.

The Imperatives for EMR Adoption

Chapter Preview:
- The economic and political pressures on healthcare are extraordinary.
- EMRs are a critical component of healthcare infrastructure.
- Adopting an EMR will improve the organization's quality of care, patient safety and efficiency.
- Adopting an EMR early gives the organization a competitive advantage.

" *There are risks and costs to a program of action, but they are far less than the long-range risks and costs of comfortable inaction.*"

~ John F. Kennedy

The economic and political pressures on healthcare are extraordinary

The most durable tools are created through the process of forging rather than casting. Using extreme heat and compression, metal is subjected to tremendous stress as it is shaped. Ironically, this tremendous stress is what actually creates the strength in the tool. Casting, on the other hand, is a fairly stress free process in which the metal is simply poured into a mold and left to harden. As a result, it is brittle, and therefore not as valuable in terms of strength and resiliency as a forged metal product. Consider the application of this metaphor to the state of healthcare today. Through tremendous economic, political and consumer-driven stress, healthcare is literally being forged into a stronger and more resilient shape.

> "Through tremendous economic, political and consumer-driven stress, healthcare is literally being forged into a stronger and more resilient shape."

We are experiencing the toughest economic times this nation has seen since the Great Depression. For nearly 50 years, healthcare costs in the United States have climbed at an alarming rate. Between 1960 and 2000, total healthcare expenditures as a percentage of gross domestic product (GDP) have nearly tripled and show no signs of slowing (Organisation for Economic Co-operation and Development, 2008.) (See Figure 2.1).

Figure 2.1: Total Expenditures on Health as a Percentage of GDP in the United States

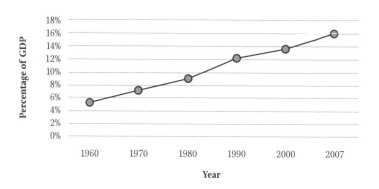

Today we spend approximately 17 percent of our GDP on healthcare, making it the largest single sector of the economy, and this number is projected to reach 20 percent by 2017 (National Coalition on Health Care, 2009). Yet physicians are working harder for declining or flat reimbursement from both public and private payers. In sharp contrast to other professionals, physicians' net income from the practice of medicine declined about 7 percent between 1995 and 2003 (after adjusting for inflation), according to a national study by the Center for Studying Health System Change (Tu, 2006). The average number of hours worked by physicians for all medically related activities in 2003 was 53.2 hours per week (Parapundit.com, 2006). These forces are creating economic, political and social pressures on our industry that will inevitably change the shape of healthcare. It is up to us to ensure the result is a stronger, more resilient healthcare system.

On February 17, 2009, the American Recovery and Reinvestment Act (ARRA) provided financial incentives to the field of Health Information Technology to make significant progress toward nationwide EMR adoption. The ARRA allocated $59 billion to the improvement of healthcare, including health IT, primary care physician training, chronic disease research, community health centers and research, and just over $19 billion in net appropriations for The Health Information Technology for Economic and Clinical Health Act (HITECH). According to the legislation, the HITECH Act aims to spur the widespread adoption of health information technology and enable electronic exchange of health information. For our industry, the HITECH Act gives us an opportunity to change the game completely by providing both the financial incentive and sense of urgency to make EMR adoption a priority.

Let's begin with the financial incentives. Although the net appropriation for the HITECH Act is about $19 billion, the government expects to spend $38 billion on this

> "the HITECH Act gives us an opportunity to change the game completely by providing both the financial incentive and sense of urgency to make EMR adoption a priority."

portion of the stimulus. The net appropriation assumes a savings of at least $18.5 billion as a result of the projected penalties and savings. The incentives encompass both Medicare and Medicaid.

Figure 2.2 illustrates the incentives for physicians.

Figure 2.2: Medicaid & Medicare Reimbursements

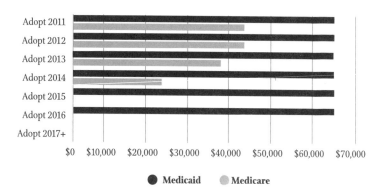

Hospital-based physicians are not eligible for individual incentive payments, but their institutions are eligible, and the incentives are enticing. For hospitals, the potential revenue starts at $2 million per year – adult money! The Medicare incentives send a strong message: the earliest adopters receive more money and those who don't adopt will be penalized. Adopting an EMR by 2011/2012 means that each physician receives up to $44,000; waiting to adopt until 2014 lowers the amount each physician receives by half – to $24,000. Waiting until 2015 will cause the annual Medicare reimbursement to decrease by 1% to 3% in subsequent years. In the past, the lack of funding for EMR adoption was one of the chief barriers for organizations. This legislation clearly begins to address that barrier.

EMRs are a critical component
of healthcare infrastructure

Both universal adoption of EMRs and interoperability are required to forge a more efficient and effective healthcare system. The Office of the National Coordinator (ONC) for Health Information Technology is tasked with creating a nationwide interoperable health information network to provide a secure infrastructure to connect healthcare providers and consumers (Nationwide Health Information Network, 2009). This is a mammoth undertaking requiring oversight of everything from privacy and security to establishment of standards and certification processes, but a worthy cause considering the potential benefits.

A secure, interoperable health record, available to a patient anywhere in the country, depends on every clinician adopting an EMR. How might this vision directly benefit the organization?

- Imagine the hours and frustration saved in hunting down paper charts, missing laboratory and imaging reports and other loose paper
- Imagine never treating a patient again without full knowledge of allergies, medications and previous medical history
- Imagine managing the care of chronically-ill patients with automatic screening reminders and evidence-based medicine guidelines
- Imagine having a complete medical record available when covering for another physician's patients
- Imagine the ease of participating in insurers' pay for perfor-

mance programs and other quality initiatives
- Imagine the decrease in medication errors and time savings for physicians with electronic prescribing

EMRs will transform healthcare by providing clinicians access to comprehensive medical information that is secure, standardized and shared. Specifically they promote increased healthcare quality, error prevention, reduced healthcare costs and increased efficiency. To achieve these benefits, the EMR must encompass certain functionality. Our study suggests most organizations do some "picking and choosing" among the available EMR functionalities when they implement a system. This customization can accelerate adoption, but it can also lead to an EMR that is little more valuable than a paper chart. In many cases, the more functionality the organization adopts, the more value they achieve, especially in the Clinical Decision Support (CDS) and order entry management realms. DesRoches et al conducted a national study of 2758 physicians, to determine the proportion of physicians using EMR records in an office setting (DesRoches et al, 2008). Their work provided evidence of the rate of implementation and defined both a basic and a fully functional EMR. Figure 2.3 illustrates that the full EMR includes some of the most challenging functionalities for physicians, yet these are essential to improving quality of care.

> "EMRs will transform healthcare by providing clinicians access to comprehensive medical information that is secure, standardized and shared."

If an organization is tempted to forego their adoption of critical functionality just to avoid physician resistance, they should immediately revisit their business case for implementing an EMR. Allowing fears of user resistance to drive these decisions will quickly diminish the value of the application.

Figure 2.3: Basic vs. Full Use of an EMR/EHR

Basic	Full
• Recording patient clinical and demographic data	• Recording patient clinical and demographic data including medical history and follow-up
• Order entry for prescriptions	• Fully functional order entry management (includes ordering prescriptions, ordering laboratory tests and radiology tests, and orders and prescriptions sent electronically)
• Viewing laboratory and imaging results	• Viewing laboratory and imaging results including electronic images returned
	• Clinical decision support including drug interactions and contraindications, out-of-range test levels highlighted, reminders for guideline-based interventions or screenings.

Adopting an EMR will improve the organization's quality of care, patient safety and efficiency

We have the opportunity to transform healthcare by providing clinicians and consumers access to comprehensive medical information that is secure, standardized and shared. A growing body of literature confirms the value of EHRs in improving patient safety, improving coordination of care, enhancing documentation, reducing administrative inefficiencies, facilitating clinical decision-making and adherence to evidence-based clinical guidelines (Chen et al, 2009). We will not spend time on a comprehensive literature review here, but we have included a summary of some of the most compelling literature in Appendix A to illustrate the evidence for improved outcomes.

A healthy dose of skepticism will serve us well as we review the EMR literature, not because it is misleading, but because it doesn't tell the whole story. Considering the strong evidence for EMRs, why haven't more organizations implemented them? Only 17% of physician practices report use of an EMR (DesRoches et al, 2008). Why did we begin this book with a story of unsatisfactory adoption and outcomes? Why do we continue to hear stories of user resistance, software that isn't ready for prime time, workflow struggles, higher than expected costs and lower than expected revenues, increases in staffing and worse quality metrics? The disconnect between the evidence in the literature and our real-world experiences is borne in the assumption that implementing an EMR and adopting an EMR are synonymous.

Adopting an EMR early gives the organization a competitive advantage

We are living in an era that is a critical turning point in Health Information Technology. We have the technology, legislation, funding, resources and sense of urgency to make a giant leap in how we apply technology to healthcare. Yet, according to Gladwell's definition, we haven't reached the tipping point – that magic moment when an idea, trend, or social behavior crosses a threshold, tips, and spreads like wildfire (Gladwell, 2002). Many of us are waiting, waiting to hear more details on meaningful use, waiting to understand the logistics for the funding and incentives, waiting to see how it goes for someone else, waiting to wait. For those willing to seize the opportunity, now is the time to break away.

> "We have the technology, legislation, funding, resources and sense of urgency to make a giant leap in how we apply technology to healthcare."

Let's consider another metaphor. The mile run is a grueling track and field race that can easily be used as a metaphor to articulate a "breakaway;" an advantage created by purposely sprinting away from the group at a point when all runners are experiencing the greatest pain. Halfway through the notorious four-lap race, at the beginning of the third lap, the breakaway occurs. Up to this point, nearly all runners are still tightly packed together, jockeying for position, cruising at a pace that pushes each runner's pulse to between 160 and 190 beats per minute. Lactic acid is accumulating in the large leg muscles, lungs burn as they are filled to capacity and emptied every second, and each runner's brain constantly takes stock of the body's condition even as it craves oxygen for itself. At this point, every runner in the pack must make a very tough decision: to summon a burst of speed and attempt to win by breaking away from the other runners, or to let others go ahead and rationalize that winning is not really so important.

The breakaway is more than a physical action; it is the most significant mental challenge a runner faces. The runner must put all bodily pain and mental anguish aside if they are to break away and win. The breakaway lasts only 20 to 30 seconds, but it is devastating for those who choose to avoid it, and inspiring for those who choose to go faster and become part of the lead pack. The leaders move continuously ahead of those left behind, drawing strength from the exhilarating sensation of actually being in a position to win. Their attention is focused outward, toward the future, on reaching the finish line first. Those who follow are immediately consumed by physical exhaustion and the deep disappointment of watching all opportunity for victory vanish. Their attention is focused inward, toward the past, on wondering why they didn't have the strength to stay with the leaders.

A similar phenomenon will occur in healthcare as many organizations compete in a relatively equal position of market share and growth, with comparable equipment and technological sophistication. Suddenly, one organization chooses to make a significant move to change the way they practice by rapidly adopting an EMR, leaving their competitors behind. Just like the runner who initiates the break-

> "Suddenly, one organization chooses to make a significant move to change the way they practice by rapidly adopting an EMR, leaving their competitors behind."

away, a healthcare organization that quickly sets itself apart from its competitors becomes outwardly focused on winning. People in these organizations, especially clinicians, are typically more patient-centered, have higher morale and understand how their daily contribution fits into the overall competitive plan. Conversely, organizations that have fallen behind tend to focus on all the internal issues that put them in a losing position. They typically engage in cost-reduction measures, technology avoidance and discrediting those perceived to be responsible for the deteriorating performance. These are the companies that will continually seek the quick fix.

Our research supports the notion that a breakaway is initiated when organizations decide to invest not just in technology, but in the people, processes and outcomes that can truly change healthcare. Technology alone does not solve problems, but with the right investment in people and process, it can drive change. For decades, HIT has been plodding forward, but we can no longer tolerate this slow pace. The HITECH Act creates the sense of urgency we need to build the infrastructure and processes to truly change the game of healthcare. By waiting, we risk losing money through the HITECH Act penalties, but more importantly, we risk losing the opportunity to make a bold move to achieve a higher level of patient care, quality and safety that this technology promotes.

> "Our research supports the notion that a breakaway is initiated when organizations decide to invest not just in technology, but in the people, processes and outcomes that can truly change healthcare."

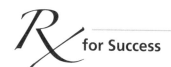 for Success

- Come to terms with the stress related to the adoption of an EMR and recognize that it will create a stronger and more resilient solution.
- Take advantage of the undeniable financial and clinical incentives of adopting an EMR today.
- Reap the benefits of a secure, standardized and shared EMR.
- Break away from competitors by being an early adopter of EMR.

Why Implementation Is Not Adoption

Chapter Preview:

- Implementation and adoption of an EMR are not synonymous. To achieve improved outcomes, adoption is mandatory.
- Moving from an EMR implementation focus to an EMR adoption focus requires a significant overhaul in how we think, how we lead, and how we behave.
- Our research presents a methodology for lasting EMR adoption.

" "The innovation-decision process can lead to either adoption, *a decision to make full use of an innovation* as the best course of action available, or rejection, a decision not to adopt an innovation.""

~ Everett M. Rogers

Diffusion of Innovations, 5th Ed., 1995

34

I t was 8 pm on a Friday evening, and the administrator of a 12-physician primary care practice sighed heavily as he reflected on the past six months. Their group had completed two successful go-live events in less than three months. By the end of the first quarter, each ambulatory site was running an EMR. Although it had not been pain-free, he felt like the implementation had gone smoothly. They had been strategic in choosing a vendor, involved the right staff in the application build, offered training to staff, and provided a great deal of support through go-live.

Today, only three months later, it felt like the entire project was spiraling out of control. Physicians were frustrated by the time required to enter information, and several had even threatened to leave. A system audit indicated the creation of generic user names and passwords that clinicians were sharing, several nurses had documented potentially life-threatening errors they felt were a result of improper use of the new system, and to top it off, the upcoming executive committee meeting included a presentation on expected outcomes from the EMR.

How does a successful implementation result in poor adoption? Easily! When decision-makers focus on just one event, a successful go-live, it is very easy to forego the processes that ensure adoption. Too many organizational leaders still believe that once the application goes live, users will embrace it. However, it becomes strikingly obvious after a go-live when the key elements of adoption have been left out. Many organizations have implemented an EMR, but very few have successfully adopted the EMR.

> ● ● ● **Implementation and adoption of an** ● ● ●
> **EMR are not synonymous. To achieve improved**
> **outcomes, adoption is mandatory.**

The terms *implementation* and *adoption* are often used interchangeably, but the outcomes from them are very different. Research suggests that implementation happens as soon as the application becomes available, but that adoption happens when the organization is using the application for clinical benefit (Jha et al, 2006). Another publication suggests that implementation happens when the organization "possesses" the application, while adoption happens when they actually use it (Florida Medical Quality Assurance Physician Practice Project, 2005-2008). Because it is critical to understand how organizations fail at EMR adoption, we will take this concept one step further.

> **"Implementation happens when the EMR goes live, essentially after a successful switch "on" of the application. Adoption is a dynamic process that requires a sustained effort for the life of the application."**

Implementation happens when the EMR goes live, essentially after a successful switch "on" of the application. Adoption is a dynamic process that requires a sustained effort for the life of the application.

36

A good indicator of a high level of adoption is when everyone is using the EMR according to the organization's prescribed policies and procedures, or best practices. Adoption enables an organization to achieve the outcomes described in the literature: improved quality, safety and efficiency, and ultimately a positive return on investment.

We first recognized the differences in outcomes between organizations who focus on implementation and those that focus on adoption as a result of our interviews with large physician practice groups. We learned that the gap between perceived adoption of an EMR and actual use of the application is more common than we expected and is often overlooked as the organization struggles to understand the mediocre (and sometimes poor) outcomes from their EMR implementation.

Our experience and research has helped us understand the key differences between implementation and adoption. The following are indicators that adoption is at risk:

- A singular focus, by those charged with the implementation, on the go-live event
- Information Technology executive (IT) as the primary owner of the EMR project
- Lack of a clearly defined governance structure to sustain the EMR
- Disengaged leadership; leaders view the effort as compulsory and not transformational
- Clinicians are rarely involved or are resistant, especially those in formal or informal leadership roles

- An institutional belief that implementation or go-live is the final step in the process.
- No sustainable strategy to educate and engage the end users to effectively utilize the new workflow
- Lack of metrics to assess adoption and ultimately achieve projected clinical and financial outcomes
- Lack of planning for post go-live workflow changes, end-user education, metrics, and overall optimization

Moving from an EMR implementation focus to an EMR adoption focus requires a significant overhaul in how we think, how we lead, and how we behave. Figure 3.1 illustrates the fundamental differences in how leaders approach a project-based implementation versus adoption. Adoption is a dynamic process focused on outcomes. When clinicians make the system their own, the reasons for utilizing the EMR outweigh the reasons to resist it. Quality of care, safety and other important clinical metrics become considerably more important than the project schedule and go-live activities. Additionally, this clinical ownership allows an executive to focus on the business issues and financial metrics. These changes "at the top" influence end user attitude and the value of investing in educating. It also ensures that sustainment is not left to chance; it is a primary focus of the

> "Moving from an EMR implementation focus to an EMR adoption focus requires a significant overhaul in how we think, how we lead, and how we behave."

overall effort because the clinical and financial outcomes depend on it.

Figure 3.1: Implementation vs. Adoption™

	Implementation	Adoption
Emphasis	Go-live (Event)	Outcomes (Process)
Ownership	Technical/ IT	Clinical/ Executive
Success Criteria	Technological Integrity	Role-based performance
Management Focus	Project Milestones & Cost	Quality of Care
Workflow Expectations	Repair	Redesign
Clinical Involvement	Negligible	Critical
End User Attitude	Apathetic or prejudiced	Adaptable
Metrics	Project Milestones	Outcomes
Training design	Demonstrate feature & function	Role-based Simulation, task completion
Sustainment post Go-live	Left to Chance	Primary Management Focus

Our primary argument that implementation is not adoption grew out of our research, as did the solution for lasting adoption. The adoption of an EMR is highly dependent on four components: engaged leadership, proficient end users, measurement of clinical and financial outcomes, and a plan to sustain the effort for the life of the application. The components can be illustrated in a simple graphic that represents the four corners of adoption (see Figure 3.2). Although we like the simplicity of this

> "The adoption of an EMR is highly dependent on four components: engaged leadership, proficient end users, measurement of clinical and financial outcomes, and a plan to sustain the effort for the life of the application."

diagram, it does not really do the model justice. As we continue into the next four chapters, we build the model, illustrate how it operates, and demonstrate how the components integrate to form a real solution to the problem of adoption.

Figure 3.2: The Four Corners of Adoption

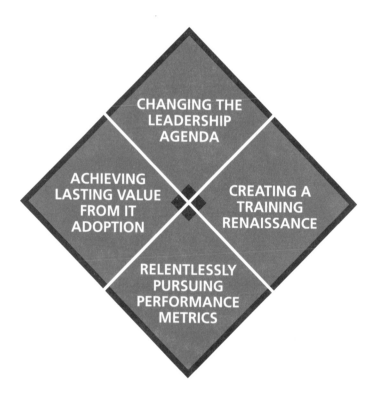

Moving from an EMR implementation focus to an EMR adoption focus requires a significant overhaul in how we think, how we lead, and how we behave.

We used the story of UTMG at the beginning of this book to illustrate the complexity of EMR adoption. The challenges are enormous and span the entire organization. Even as researchers looking in from the outside, the solutions to the problems of adoption were not immediately obvious to us. It was fairly easy to identify the recurring themes and challenges based on our research, but it was not until we were introduced to a science known as systems thinking that we began to mold a solution consistent with the ongoing and changing needs of healthcare.

In 1994, Peter Senge, a professor at MIT's Sloan School of Management, published The Fifth Discipline. Almost overnight, the book became a best seller, and Senge became famous for popularizing a science known as systems thinking. Systems thinking can help with the analysis of complex organizational problems, such as the adoption of an EMR. It is fundamentally different from traditional forms of analysis because it recognizes an inherent delay between cause and effect. Traditional event-based analysis assumes little or no delay between an event and its outcome, with the event itself scrutinized for success or failure. Event-based analysis also creates the impulse to identify the one or two issues that created a problem during the event and to direct a solution at the seemingly obvious cause.

To understand how systems thinking can help with the problem of adoption, we need to cover a few fundamentals. First of all, a reinforcing feedback process results in either a positive or negative acceleration of growth, and can be diagrammed as an archetype (Senge, 1994). An archetype is simply a diagram that tells a story. In Figure 3.3, the diagram for a positive reinforcing process is straightforward: consider the positive effect of beginning an exercise program and the improved mental and physical health that drives increased energy and reinforces exercise on subsequent days. Contrast this in Figure 3.4 with the effect of skipping one or more workouts, then feeling less fit and having less energy, resulting in skipping more workouts. This describes a negative reinforcing process.

Figure 3.3: The Positive Reinforcing Process of Exercise

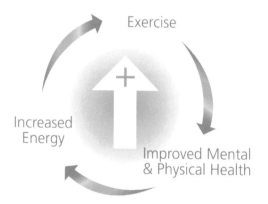

Figure 3.4: The Negative Reinforcing Process of Exercise

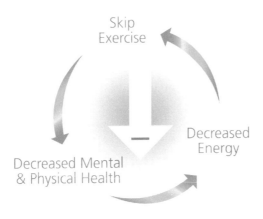

Many feedback processes contain delays between actions and their consequences (Senge, 1994). For example, it takes approximately 20 minutes for our stomachs to relay messages to our brains that we are full. When we are very hungry, we tend to eat so quickly that we completely overshoot the "full" response and end up feeling "stuffed". The inevitable delay between cause and effect in this feedback process leads us to overeat.

In relation to EMR adoption, feedback process delays may cause us to react with quick fixes that magnify the problem. Too often, we react to the problem of EMR adoption by coming up with solutions that only address the symptoms of the problem, leaving the problem itself unchanged or even worse. "Solutions that address only the symptoms of a problem, not the fundamental causes, tend to have short-term benefits at best." (Senge, 1994). Physician resistance, errors and security breaches are all symptoms of the bigger problem. If the problem is poor end user adoption of the EMR, quick-fix solutions will not be effective. Quick fixes such as blaming physicians, vendors or leaders, purchasing a new or upgraded application, forcing user compliance and ignoring poor outcomes also bring unintended consequences that actually cause a negative reinforcing feedback, further delaying the solution of the problem. Identifying the root problems and employing sustainable solutions is the only way out of the quick fix cycle. We will illustrate how the key drivers of adoption work together as a system using archetypes.

44

Our research represents a methodology for lasting EMR adoption

Based on the findings of our research, we developed a model that represents the four critical components of EMR adoption and how they work together. The diagram in Figure 3.5 (page 46) uses Senge's approach to explain the interaction among the components of the model for EMR adoption. The foundation of sustainable adoption is engaged leadership, which sits at the center of the model. Developing a strategy for long-term adoption and establishing governance begins with engaged leadership. Engaged leadership will make or break the entire effort. As our research has shown, the second driver is an effective education and training program that results in proficient end users. Proficient clinicians and staff are a result of engaged leaders, so the model builds to the right of engaged leaders. Engaged leaders and proficient users produce desired clinical and financial outcomes, and they ensure the sustainment of these outcomes long-term. The sustainment loop is a balancing loop, which is

"Based on the findings of our research, we developed a model that represents the four critical components of EMR adoption and how they work together."

a critical component of the model because it ensures that the three reinforcing loops continue to move in a positive direction. Metrics serve as the "vital signs" for adoption over time, which reinforces the work being done by leaders and end users. In the next four chapters, we will dissect the model and take a deep dive into each of these areas to demonstrate how they integrate into a sustainable solution for EMR adoption.

45

Figure 3.5: Sustainable Solution to EMR Adoption

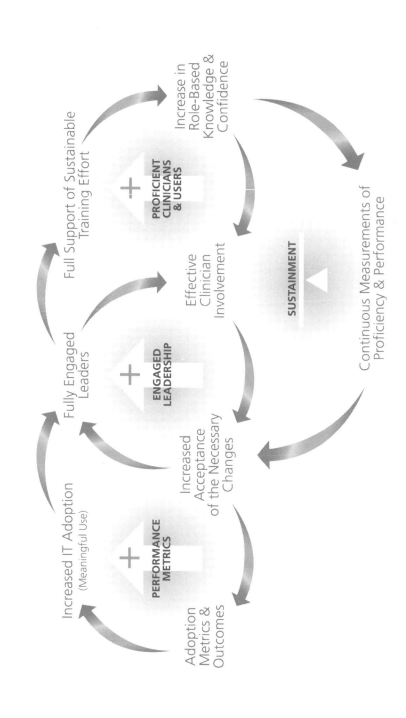

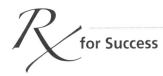

for Success

- Change your thinking regarding adoption to move beyond go-live myopia.
- Find a way to articulate the difference between implementation and adoption.
- Consider the long-term consequences of your decisions. Specifically resist quick fix decisions that won't lead to end-user adoption.
- Find the courage to end the focus on implementation and to begin a journey toward adoption.

47

48

CHAPTER FOUR

Changing the Leadership Agenda

Chapter Preview: A new leadership agenda focused on leading EMR adoption:

- Develop a Stop Doing List
- Create a Tone at the Top in the organization
- Connect to the clinical leadership
- Empower the decision makers and define their sphere of influence
- Relentlessly pursue meaningful clinical and financial impact

" *"What you do speaks so loud that I cannot hear what you say."*"

~ Ralph Waldo Emerson

Remembered for leading the Transcendentalist

movement of the early 19th century

Strewn across the dry-erase board were key words and phrases from a lively discussion with a group of respected healthcare CIOs: physician resistance; improper workflow design; ineffective training; lack of engagement; few clinical outcomes; vendor apathy; prohibitive expense. These were the most common responses to our question, "What is the most significant barrier to physician adoption of EMRs?" Initially, all of these themes seemed both relevant and equivalent in terms of identifying the barriers to EMR adoption. We talked to many bright individuals with years of healthcare and IT experience; yet many of them were still struggling in the effort to implement and adopt an EMR. Little did we know that one of these themes would trump all others as the greatest inhibitor to successful adoption of EMRs. In fact, as we would discover through our interviews, this one factor alone outweighed all other elements combined as we identified requirements for sustainable adoption of an EMR.

Our discovery came as we started to question which factors were early drivers of EMR adoption. True to our assumptions about the challenges of EMR adoption, many of our early predictions around workflow, training and vendor support were validated. We also

> "The one factor that formed a pattern across every single organization struggling with physician/clinician adoption of an EMR, however, was lack of engagement from those chosen to lead the overall effort."

verified that application vendors develop tools, but have limited time and expertise to tackle the breadth of areas required for lasting adoption. The one factor that formed a pattern across every single organization struggling with physician/clinician adoption of an EMR, however, was lack of engagement from those chosen to lead the overall effort. For many reasons, this is a hard pill to swallow. First, it places responsibility back at the feet of the earliest champions: those who decided to fund and move the entire organization forward with the implementation of the EMR. Second, it requires an already overworked executive team to make adoption a daily priority; effective leadership is an antecedent to adoption.

There is no greater barrier to adoption of a complex IT application in an ever-changing healthcare environment than believing we can simply pile this effort on top of all the other priorities and expect that we will be successful. Organizations that have disconnected, part-time and or overworked leaders at the helm of an EMR effort will struggle and may never fully adopt it. In contrast, organizations that have leaders who are fully invested in the daily march toward adoption will not only reach the early stages of adoption, but will enjoy the reinforcement of meaningful clinical and financial outcomes. To succeed in moving the people of an organization to-

> **"There is no greater barrier to adoption of a complex IT application in an ever-changing healthcare environment than believing we can simply pile this effort on top of all the other priorities and expect that we will be successful."**

ward adoption of an EMR, leaders must change the way they previously approached implementations. Their first priority must be to establish a new leadership agenda, which will create a reinforcing set of behaviors that begin the movement toward end user adoption.

> "Their first priority must be to establish a new leadership agenda, which will create a reinforcing set of behaviors that begin the movement toward end user adoption."

As we discussed in Chapter 3, leadership sits at the center of our model for lasting adoption. Leaders are in a critical position because they drive the system into either a positive or negative direction. More importantly, leaders need to be fully engaged over a significant period of time to maintain a positive reinforcing loop. Figure 4.1 (page 54) illustrates how engaged leaders ensure clinician involvement and ultimately drive increased acceptance of the changes necessary for EMR adoption.

Figure 4.1: Adoption Model - Engaged Leadership

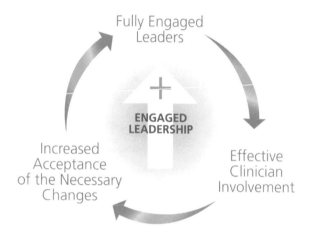

We carefully chose the term engaged to best describe the actions and behaviors required of leaders, and to avoid the negative connotation often associated with the term change management. Figure 4.2 illustrates a word map of terms related to the term engaged; interestingly, these terms also represent how engaged leaders describe their behavior on any given day as they interact with people, establish priorities and make decisions (THINKMAP Visual Thesaurus, 2010). It is engaged leaders who choose to see their roles and priorities differently and who ultimately lead their organization successfully through change.

Figure 4.2: Word Map for the Term "Engaged"

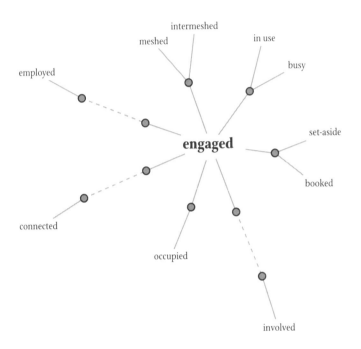

Develop a Stop Doing List

As stated earlier, the greatest barrier to adoption of a complex IT application in an ever-changing healthcare environment is the belief that we can successfully heap this effort onto a long list of other priorities. Establishing a new leadership agenda requires freeing up time for those leading the effort. Without reprioritizing leaders' daily actions, all other actions are subject to inadequate time and attention. Jim Collins, the author of *Good to Great*, popularized the concept of the Stop Doing List. In his book, he contends that one of the commonalities of companies who are able to propel themselves from being just good to being great is that they all examined everything they were currently doing and then consciously decided to stop working on some things, even major things. In his recent interview with TIME Magazine, he is even more aggressive on this topic, arguing that many companies that have recently failed have done so because they simply had too many strategic initiatives in play (TIME, 2009). His new book, *How the Mighty Fall*, centers on this topic. He contends that these initiatives literally choked the growth of the organization due to lackluster performance in many areas and stellar performance in none.

Leaders currently in charge of EMR adoption need to develop a ferocious understanding of what they are going to stop doing, and then maintain the courage to follow through on their decisions. Because it demonstrates active commitment to end users who are affected by the new workflows, this may be the single greatest action toward successful adoption of an EMR.

> **"Leaders currently in charge of EMR adoption need to develop a ferocious understanding of what they are going to stop doing, and then maintain the courage to follow through on their decisions."**

Even though we cannot prescribe specific changes to leaders' priorities, we have identified some rules based on our experience with those who have succeeded:

1. Time is one of the most valuable resources among leadership and providers. Identify the most time-consuming projects and prioritize them using the following criteria:
   - Projects/meetings that do not directly affect quality of care or safety
   - Projects/meetings that are not related to compliance or legal risk
   - Projects that can be delayed with little overall impact
   - Meetings that can be eliminated or consolidated

2. Be courageous: stop doing or postpone enough projects to enable the leadership team to declare EMR adoption as one of their top three priorities.

3. Openly communicate decisions to delay other projects throughout the organization. This provides the foundation message from leadership that EMR adoption is critical to the organization's mission. We have witnessed celebration, disbelief and clinicians' open arms when this has been done well.

4. Identify a governance method to ensure that new initiatives do not creep back into the list of priorities and consume the precious new time. We have seen great progress in stopping projects and meetings, only to find new projects and meetings sneaking in to take their place.

Create a Tone at the Top
of the organization

One of the most challenging aspects of leading the adoption of an EMR is transforming the project into a compelling and meaningful effort for everyone in the organization. When people, especially providers, believe in the cause, they will go to extraordinary lengths to ensure a successful outcome. This transformation creates and reinforces their commitment to the long-term goals of the effort.

Creating a message with purpose and constancy is not easy, and sustaining the message is even more difficult. When leaders create a tone that permeates the EMR adoption message, it will often overcome the imperfect delivery of messages shared among the end users, helping to maintain the momentum behind the effort.

In a recent conversation with pianist, composer and recording artist Kevin Asbjornson, he described the difference between a piano's tune and tone. We can draw an analogy from having multiple leaders tell the EMR adoption story. Tuning is the adjustment of a piano's strings to the correct pitch, ensuring notes played in octaves or chords will sound in harmony. Tuning is the organizational equivalent of how we connect people with equipment and

> "One of the most challenging aspects of leading the adoption of an EMR is transforming the project into a compelling and meaningful effort for everyone in the organization."

workflow. By contrast, the quality of the sound comes from adjusting the piano's tone. When the piano's tone is matched with the passion of the pianist, pure music radiates from the instrument.

Telling a powerful story of transformation through EMR adoption is the pure music that helps employees support the effort by addressing their biggest concerns. When leaders answer the big questions, like how the adoption of an EMR advances the mission of the organization, or how the changes will directly affect end users, employees are more likely to respond positively. The ultimate impact from the tone depends on providing compelling answers to these questions, but also on leader willingness and ability to make the message personal and transparent as they engage in dialogue about the changes. We have seen this effort unlock significant energy within those originally ambivalent about the effort.

There are myriad ways to develop the music from the leaders of the organization. The technique below represents a framework to develop the tone and to keep it resonating for years to come:

- The "Tone at the top" requires a rigor similar to a marketing effort replete with a value proposition that connects to the mission of the organization.
- As with any respectable marketing program, a "brand" should be developed that delivers a symbolic moniker that will have lasting recognition for the adoption life cycle. Remember, this is not an event, but rather a process that will need definition.
- Keep in mind that the "tone" requires a constant rhythm from the leaders of the organization, and rhythm comes

from a tempo of planned activities and communication efforts.

- Leaders must be visible and able to articulate the value proposition at any moment. Authenticity is the key ingredient in the message. Rather than creating new meetings, find a way to tap into current assemblies and gatherings.
- Build the "tone" into current employee feedback systems – or create a new one. Getting planned and periodic feedback from a cross-functional representation of the staff is part of the overall process to keep the rhythm. Be prepared to modify the process if the message is not making an impact.

• • • Connect to the clinical leadership • • •

Physician adoption of the EMR is critically important to an organization for four reasons:

1. Physicians choose to bring their patients to the organization, often in preference to a competitor
2. Physicians personally provide and direct patient care, thus driving revenue and cost
3. Physicians are influential with colleagues and staff because of the informal organizational power derived from their medical knowledge and expertise, and from the trust and respect they are afforded
4. Physicians can be strong supporters or detractors of the EMR through the subtle exercise of this power

The key to physician adoption is physician engagement. This engagement must occur at several levels. The first is at the governance level, through a physician body or council. A charter should formally establish the council, delineating the membership and often including representatives from all clinical departments. It is important to include EMR supporters as well as "curmudgeons". In most cases, the council chair should be a practicing physician and the CMO/CMIO and CIO should be staff to the council. The council should construct a vision statement that describes the benefits the EMR will provide to patients, physicians, staff and the organization. The responsibilities and accountabilities of the council should be clearly explained in the charter; they often include specific policies, procedures and best practices for physician use of the EMR. Finally, and most importantly, the top leadership of the organization must formally endorse and empower the council to carry out its responsibilities.

> **"The key to physician adoption is physician engagement."**

The next levels of engagement are at the individual physician level. The council members should act as advocates for the EMR with their departmental colleagues. It can be very helpful to have several physician champions - individuals who are widely respected and well-networked within the organization. They do not have to be technology "nerds", and they often benefit from having at least a sprinkling of gray hair. Physician super-users who are highly proficient in the use of the EMR can be valuable resources as at-the-

61

> "A high level of physician engagement can overcome or ameliorate the common barriers to physician adoption, including resistance to abandoning the paper chart, the investment of time required to learn the new system and the initial drop in productivity until the user attains proficiency."

elbow support for their colleagues and as mentors for new physicians.

A high level of physician engagement can overcome or ameliorate the common barriers to physician adoption, including resistance to abandoning the paper chart, the investment of time required to learn the new system and the initial drop in productivity until the user attains proficiency. Growing evidence from studies in the literature indicates that the use of CPOE, medication management and CDS functionalities result in improved patient care quality and safety. And the latter, after all, is the raison d'être for healthcare providers.

• • • Empower the decision makers and • • • define their sphere of influence

Implementing an EMR requires thoughtful consideration of the policies and procedures that will govern the use of the system. There are many stakeholders with a myriad of opinions and often competing interests that can dramatically slow adoption of the EMR. Adherence to a well-defined governance process ensures that the right people are involved at the right time with the right information. The lack of governance allows the wrong people to debate decisions endlessly, ignore standards easily and often conclude by making the wrong decisions. Leaders must establish strong governance processes to define expectations around adoption of the new application, involve the right stakeholders to make decisions, establish policies and best practices and ultimately evaluate performance against expectations. Governance should also be flexible enough to evolve over time. The governance needed during an implementation may be very different from the governance needed two years after go-live. In our experience, very few organizations appreciate the significance of governance in adoption of an EMR.

Most organizations develop policies, procedures and best practices, but rarely measure their usage. We have all worked in organizations where significant time was spent on establishing best practices only to find very few people actually observing them. This lack of accountability weakens the governance process. Effective governance closes the loop by monitoring actual adoption in end user work product. This creates a dynamic process that can evolve over time to meet the needs of the organization.

"Effective governance closes the loop by monitoring actual adoption in end user work product. This creates a dynamic process that can evolve over time to meet the needs of the organization."

Relentlessly pursue meaningful clinical and financial impact

The payoff for adopting an EMR comes in the form of clinical and financial outcomes. If results are neither tracked nor realized, the effort is truly a waste of time and money. Our expectations need to be realistic, but ultimately it is the leaders who are accountable for relentlessly pursuing the tracking of outcomes.

When we conducted the interviews for our research, we were shocked at the lack of clinical and financial metrics being collected, especially considering the effort and money invested. In many cases, tracking metrics was simply not a high priority. The data was available, but the process for collecting, analyzing and reporting on the data was missing. The time and resources had not been spent to obtain the story that the data could tell.

Since most people would agree that outcomes are critically important to gauging the success of an EMR adoption, their measurement must be part of the new leadership agenda. Leaders must incent the right people to collect, analyze and report on the data. Similar to engaging clinicians, this takes some finesse. The good news is that clinicians are generally interested in these metrics and may be more compliant with use of the EMR if they understand the clinical and financial goals. We usually suggest identifying a few key metrics that are easy to collect and that will be of interest to the clinicians.

> "If results are neither tracked nor realized, the effort is truly a waste of time and money."

Once those metrics are published, it does not take long to find the data enthusiasts in the organization and engage them in more sophisticated reporting. These metrics are the key to optimizing use of the system, achieving highly engaged end users and ultimately improving patient care.

The new leadership agenda for EMR adoption requires a significant change in how we lead. Newton's First Law of Motion states "An object at rest tends to stay at rest and an object in motion tends to stay in motion with the same speed and in the same direction, unless acted upon by an unbalanced force." This is an important concept to consider as we ask clinicians to change the way they practice medicine. We all have a strong tendency to keep doing what we're doing. In fact, it is our natural tendency to resist changes. In physics, this tendency to resist changes is called inertia. In healthcare, inertia represents the status quo. EMR adoption represents significant change to the way we work, and it is natural to resist that change. However, because the benefits outweigh the pain of change in the long term, we need to find a way to overcome inertia. In physics, the only way to overcome inertia is to apply an unbalanced force. In

> "In healthcare, that unbalanced force is engaged leaders who invest themselves in the outcome and create the momentum necessary for the organization to achieve adoption of an EMR."

healthcare, that unbalanced force is engaged leaders who invest themselves in the outcome and create the momentum necessary for the organization to achieve adoption of an EMR.

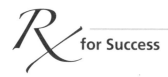

for Success

- Start today by establishing a new leadership agenda focused on EMR adoption.
- Develop a Stop Doing List that puts EMR adoption in the top three priorities.
- Create a Tone at the Top that permeates the entire organization.
- Engage and connect to clinical leadership; their support is critical for success.
- Empower the decision makers and clearly define their sphere of influence.
- Be relentless in the pursuit of meaningful clinical and financial outcomes.

Creating a Training Renaissance

Chapter Preview:
- "The definition of insanity is doing the same thing over and over and expecting different results."
  – Benjamin Franklin
- Traditional training methods are a disservice to clinicians; they are slow, expensive and ineffective.
- We need a training renaissance to help clinicians learn new technology fast.
- Proficient and confident end users are the most valuable asset in achieving and maintaining adoption.

"The definition of insanity is doing the same thing over and over and expecting different results." – Benjamin Franklin

It is amazing what some travelers attempt to bring on an airplane. On one of our research trips, we followed a woman up the escalator in the airport as she schlepped enough luggage to equip four people. Coincidentally, this same woman was seated between us on the flight. Apparently, she had been forced to check her largest bag, but was adamant about carrying on three others.

During the flight, we observed her wrestle with four bulging three-ring binders, placing sticky notes on specific pages and jotting down reminders in the text. About an hour into the flight, we learned she was bound for New Jersey to facilitate a week-long EMR training class. Suddenly we were both more interested! We traded stories and discussed the challenges of effective EMR training. By the end of the flight, we had seen the contents of her four binders. They contained incredibly detailed information about every function of the application. Not unlike the bag she attempted to stuff into the overhead bin, she was apparently about to try to jam hundreds of hours of material into one forty-hour training session.

Traditional vendor training often follows this exact scenario, packing an unrealistic amount of content into marathon training sessions. Delays in the application build, testing and other unforeseen events force training to the last possible moment and then cram as much material and information as possible into the available time period. The train-the-trainer method amplifies the issues; imagine depending on only a few people to transfer the information to everyone in the organization - a recipe for disaster. Like the game of Telephone, information shared across multiple people loses integrity in each iteration. Train-the-trainer relies on individuals to understand, remember and clearly communicate complex information. All too often, inaccurate information is passed along. E-learning, web-based training and online learning provide consistent information, but are rarely tailored to the learner's needs and are subject to the same limitations of traditional training.

• • • Traditional training methods are a • • • disservice to clinicians; they are slow, expensive and ineffective

When organizations struggle with adoption of new technology, they often blame the end user for resisting change. Complaints about physician resistance are especially common. While it is true that user resistance can slow adoption, the term places blame directly on users instead of addressing the real problem. In truth, the user experience is simply a barometer of how prepared the organization is for change and how they have chosen to educate their users. Physician resistance is a symptom of poor training.

Speed-to-proficiency describes our goal for end users – and an effective process allows the organization to escape the endless cycle of repeating the same efforts while expecting different results. We want proficient end users who successfully and quickly learn exactly what they need to know in order to fulfill their specific role in the organization. Decision makers that short-change training are three times more likely to have their IT projects fall short of business and project goals and organizations that

> "In truth, the user experience is simply a barometer of how prepared the organization is for change and how they have chosen to educate their users. Physician resistance is a symptom of poor training."

underfund training almost guarantee that end users will have a sub-standard understanding of new systems (Aldrich, 2000; Burleson, 2001; Wheatley, 2000). Compounding the problem, physician resistance is the most familiar complaint made by organizations, while the most common physician response? "We don't have time for training and it isn't effective anyway!"

We need a training renaissance to help clinicians learn new technology fast

It is time to question the traditional training model for getting users up to speed on new technology. We know from nearly nine decades of research about adult learning that humans do not learn without a natural progression from discovery through experience. The average human brain is a very poor storage device for information and data, unless that information is recalled and reinforced immediately by experiential activities. The one-time training event stuffed with an overloaded agenda is an almost certain waste if a user does not have the opportunity to progress through the natural learning process.

> "The one-time training event stuffed with an overloaded agenda is an almost certain waste if a user does not have the opportunity to progress through the natural learning process."

Adopting an EMR is an enormous undertaking for any organization, small or large, because it touches every employee and every operational process. In the past, healthcare organizations could spend days, weeks and months training and retraining staff. Today, there is a sense of urgency to adopt an EMR faster. The HITECH Act requires organizations to prove meaningful use: use of the new system must achieve improved clinical outcomes to qualify. In addition, the faster organizations adopt, the more money they receive. This will require a radically different process focused on helping clinicians achieve proficiency by role in the new technology quickly.

Adoption is driven by a sustainable and effective learning solution for clinicians and end users. Take a look at Figure 5.1. When the organization develops a curriculum focused on end user knowledge and confidence, the outcome is proficiency. Proficiency among all users then results in effective use of the system. Understanding how clinicians are trained in medicine may provide some insight into why high levels of knowledge and confidence overcome physician resistance. Physicians resist because they have spent years honing their knowledge and experience in their fields of expertise and are now being handed a tool that they do not understand how to use and do not trust in using to treat patients. When physicians are highly knowledgeable and confident in how to use the system to treat patients, they embrace the technology instead of resisting it.

> "When physicians are highly knowledgeable and confident in how to use the system to treat patients, they embrace the technology instead of resisting it."

Figure 5.1: Adoption Model - Engaged Leadership, Proficient Clinicians & Users

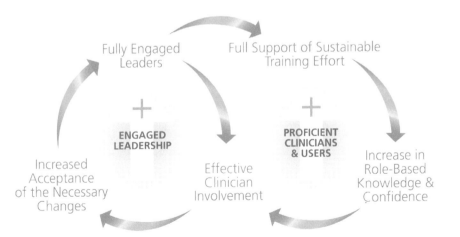

It is time to use this past century's research on human learning strategically, applying a heavy dose of common sense (Kolb, 1984). A number of steps and classifications have been used to describe the way in which a human learns and retains knowledge. We will use the aviation industry to introduce a new learning process and then apply the principles to healthcare.

In the early 1980s, the commercial airline industry faced a similar challenge to what we face in healthcare today. A breakthrough in manufacturing processes led to a dramatic decrease in the time it took to build an airplane. For the first time in history, the production of airplanes outpaced a pilot's ability to adopt the new digital avionics and flight controls. It was quite a conundrum: the conversion of the new digital avionics from the outdated analog systems made air travel safer, but pilots did not have enough time to get trained. This is analogous to physicians learning to use EMRs. Physicians and pilots have a lot in common: they receive years of specialized training in their field, they have enormous responsibility for the safety of others and they work in a complex and highly stressful environment. So why are we shocked when they refuse to attend classroom training or question the value of a train-the-trainer approach?

The commercial airline industry solved the problem by designing flight simulators that closely mimic the experience of flying an actual plane. They invented a solution that was relevant, timely, hands-on and sustainable – and that fit the pilot's needs.

Just like pilots, clinicians must advance through four learning phases to learn the new information: introduction, assimilation, translation and accumulation (Fred, 2002). In the first phase, the learner is exposed to a new set of data and recognizes that the information is different. In the second phase, the learner assimilates the new data with their own personal knowledge and experience. This is the stage in which the learner passes judgment on whether the new information or po-

> "Just like pilots, clinicians must advance through four learning phases to learn the new information: introduction, assimilation, translation and accumulation (Fred, 2002)."

tential new skill has any benefit to them. When they perceive that it does not, their active participation in the learning process is at risk. In phase three, the learner places the new information into the context of their job, showing that they understand how it fits. Without translation, the learner stops at being informed and rarely makes the leap to any form of application or practice. Phases one, two and occasionally part of three are the usual fodder for the traditional training process. In fact, nearly 60 billion dollars per year are spent on this part of the proficiency process alone (American Society of Training and Development, 2009). Sadly, without the fourth phase, the end user does not truly adopt, wasting both user time and organization resources.

It is common for organizations to rely solely on the effectiveness of phases one and two; however, the highest payoff lies in the final and most time-consuming phase. In the fourth phase, knowledge is transformed into action through an accumulation of experiences using the new knowledge in practice or application. This phase is the most critical, yet is often left to chance when organizations plan an HIT implementation. Many organizations do not appreciate the importance of the users practicing what they have learned, testing through trial and error and receiving feedback on their performance. As a result, organizations often leave this most critical of the phases unfunded. Considered a cost savings in the short term, ignoring phase four actually costs the organization more because of increased turnover and overtime, clinician resistance to change and meager improvements to clinical outcomes. Following through to phase four means shortening the cycle time to proficiency via rapid accumulation of experience, affording the best opportunity for an organization to gain significant competitive advantage.

> "Many organizations do not appreciate the importance of the users practicing what they have learned, testing through trial and error and receiving feedback on their performance."

When designed correctly, simulators literally change how healthcare providers learn new technology. First, they are designed separately for each role that will use the application. Physicians and nurses do not perform the same tasks, so a generic simulator developed for clinicians is ineffective. Individuals do not have to learn to use every function in an application, but they do have to learn all functions related to their specific role. It is a mistake to teach every function of the entire application; it overwhelms the user with extraneous information and dilutes the information that is critical to their job role. Imagine being required to learn every function of Microsoft Excel before being able to create a simple spreadsheet. Most of us would be much prefer learning only the tasks necessary to create the spreadsheet and then discovering the bells and whistles only as needed.

"When designed correctly, simulators literally change how healthcare providers learn new technology."

Consider a physician forced to attend the upcoming EMR training session planned by the woman with the overstuffed binders. He surely cannot help but question the level and depth of material planned for the week, not to mention the lost revenue from not seeing patients on those days. He knows he will attend training along with medical students and residents – posing a challenge on how all the potential scenarios could possibly be covered. If they were all asked to achieve the same level of understanding of all of the material, most of the time spent in training would be wasted on at least two-thirds of them. Common sense indicates that the target for proficiency varies greatly by role, because each role in healthcare is different. Someone in an administrative role does not require the medical proficiency of a nurse or physician. Conversely, a clinician requires only the basics of how patients are arrived in the clinic, whereas front desk staff needs to know the most detail about the processes of scheduling, arrival, registration and check out. One of the easiest, most pragmatic methods to reduce the cycle time to proficiency is to define the proficiency level required for a particular job role.

Defining the target proficiency level for performance in a particular assignment or task will take us on the shortest path to proficiency for a particular user or group of users. Beginning with the end in mind, we should always define the threshold level of proficiency before launching an elaborate system of training toward unnecessary goals.

The threshold level of proficiency is the point at which healthcare providers can collectively create and deliver value to a patient within a process (Fred, 2002).

The threshold level of proficiency is crucial to competitive advantage, for it is the point at which a user begins to contribute value to the operation in a particular job or task. For each of the varying degrees of contribution needed throughout an organization, there is a corresponding set of proficiency levels: discovery, literacy, fluency and mastery. A combination of the acquisition of new information with one's previous experience and know-how, discovery can be achieved through a formal training event, multiple forms of media, a dramatic event (e.g., safety accident) or through the grapevine. At the literacy level of proficiency, one can articulate the newly acquired information within the context of his or her job. Fluency is a function of the amount of experience accumulated over a period of time that will allow one to perform at an acceptable level of perfor-

> "The threshold level of proficiency is the point at which healthcare providers can collectively create and deliver value to a patient within a process (Fred, 2002)."

mance. Mastery is also a function of the amount of experience accumulated over a period of time, but enough experience has been gained to be considered a subject-matter expert.

By identifying the required levels of proficiency across an organization, decision-makers take the first step toward a precise strategy to help users adopt new technology. This allows them to make the best use of both time and money to achieve crucial initial performance levels. When addressed this way, for the first time, proficiency is viewed across an organization strategically instead of tactically. Resources are applied more strategically and workers begin reaching discovery and literacy levels very quickly. In addition, very few employees need to achieve mastery in their first learning efforts. Physicians, nurses, technicians, IT and administrative support employees all need varying levels of proficiency. In this example, only the super users and IT (about five percent of the total group) need to reach the mastery level as their initial threshold. The majority of the healthcare provider team only needs a fluency threshold level, and they can achieve this with a much shorter course, followed by rapid rounds of practice.

Proficient and confident end users are the most valuable asset in achieving and maintaining adoption

Software implementations often fail due to poor end user adoption. The business case for a new EMR assumes that users will learn to use the system quickly. Yet end user education is often underfunded, poorly planned and undervalued. When users cannot use the system according to prescribed workflows, the business case for the system quickly falls apart, resulting in poor clinical and financial outcomes.

> **"Software implementations often fail due to poor end user adoption."**

Traditional training methods such as train-the-trainer and classroom instruction have never been truly effective ways for end users to acquire and apply knowledge. Classroom instruction is too passive a learning experience for the user. By the time the user gets their hands on the system, they cannot remember what they learned in class. Classroom training also takes clinicians and other critical staff away from work for hours or days. Train-the-trainer methods rely heavily on expert trainers, but these individuals often lack the time, knowledge and expertise to teach effectively. Yet, in our research interviews, every organization we spoke with was still relying on these methods. Many agreed that their current training could be more effective, but most did not have the time, resources, or staff to address it.

> **"Yet end user education is often underfunded, poorly planned and undervalued."**

We had the opportunity to work with one of the world's largest diagnostic imaging centers as they implemented a Radiology Information System/Picture Archiving and Communication System (RIS/PACS) for more than 870 end users at over 60 locations. Prior to our involvement, they had utilized a train-the-trainer model. Training consisted of eight to 12 hours of lecture and demonstration at an offsite location, not including travel time of two to four hours. After users at only a few sites completed training, it was apparent that they were not adopting the system. The organization documented errors resulting from inconsistent practices and workarounds in the clinics. The errors resulted in increased insurance claim denials or delays, incorrect or incomplete patient information and increased days in accounts receivable. Based on retrospective site audits, adoption of the application never occurred because of the ineffective training, lack of retention and site-specific workflow issues. On average, it took employees 120 days (approximately 24 weeks based on a five-day work week) to achieve fluency in the application. The combination of these results led to our involvement and ultimately to a revamp of the process for educating users.

We began the new process by first engaging leadership and then developing a communication plan that involved site managers. We also performed extensive workflow analysis, capturing the current workflows and designing new workflows for each role in the organization. Users learned to perform the tasks in their role using online learning. Far from being a passive method of delivery, this online learning put the user inside simulations of real clinical scenarios. Individuals with expertise in the workflow by role then provided at-the-elbow support for users. The learning outcomes were dramatically different. The average user spent two hours practicing the key tasks in their role with the simulations. During the week of go-live, the average user was certified to use the application within four days. The time investment by the average employee was approximately four days (two hours practicing with the simulators and four days using the application during go-live week). Therefore, the average speed to proficiency was four days and the employees were actually working in the live system for all except two hours. When compared to the initial site audits, the new process produced proficient users in 4 days, compared to 120 days, returning 116 days of productivity per employee to the organization. Extrapolated across all employees, the savings add up to 101,384 days (see Figure 5.2).

Figure 5.2: Train the Trainer Versus the Adoption Model

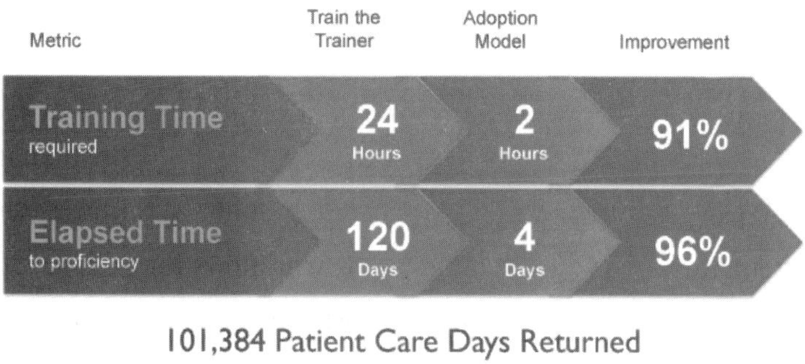

Metric	Train the Trainer	Adoption Model	Improvement
Training Time required	24 Hours	2 Hours	91%
Elapsed Time to proficiency	120 Days	4 Days	96%

101,384 Patient Care Days Returned

The pace at which learners adopt the new technology is critical, but so is the outcome of their learning. Two strong indicators of proficiency are knowledge and confidence. We developed a methodology for measuring both knowledge and confidence as indicators of proficiency. We assess end user knowledge and confidence at baseline, after the application go-live and regularly thereafter.

Consider UTMG's results. UTMG leaders knew that they had poor adoption after their initial implementation. We also recognized the signs of poor adoption based on their lack of clinical and financial outcomes, but there was no data to measure the magnitude of the problem. We immediately did a baseline assessment of user knowledge and confidence that helped UTMG quantify the problem they needed to solve. Only 66 percent of UTMG employees had an excellent or good knowledge of how to perform their tasks in the new TouchWorks application. Similarly, only 76 percent of employees had an excellent or good level of confidence in performing their tasks in the new application. We assessed the same factors after they completed the assigned simulators and found that knowledge increased from 66 to 97 percent and confidence increased from 76 to 96 percent - a dramatic and statistically significant change. However, in order to prevent erosion of these adoption results, UTMG will have to continue to measure and sustain this level of knowledge and confidence in their end users.

> "The pace at which learners adopt the new technology is critical, but so is the outcome of their learning."

Our bias for metrics has served us well. We have accumulated data on knowledge and confidence of over 2,000 healthcare providers. Our goal is to establish benchmarks for healthcare organizations striving to improve adoption of new technologies in healthcare. Today we believe a minimum of 90 percent of users must have either an excellent or good level of both knowledge and confidence in using the new technology after the initial go-live. By the end of the first year, organizations should achieve at least 95 percent on both knowledge and confidence and maintain that level for the lifetime of the application.

To achieve adoption, users need to accumulate experience in the application. Give them the opportunity to become proficient in the tasks they use to serve patients and they will quickly adopt the new technology.

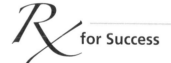 **for Success**

- Choose to train clinicians in a new way. The processes and technology exist to dramatically improve end user adoption.
- Dedicate your training effort to ensuring end users will achieve threshold proficiency.
- Create an environment where end users can practice and accumulate experience in the application using clinical scenarios.
- Require that every end user achieve high levels of proficiency, knowledge and confidence.

Relentlessly Pursuing Performance Metrics

Chapter Preview:
- Adoption is a prerequisite for meaningful use and we must measure it.
- The first indicator of adoption is end user proficiency.
- Performance metrics, the clinical and financial outcomes, demonstrate the value of adoption.
- Performance metrics drive the organization to optimize use of the EMR.

"*Trying to improve something when you don't have a means of measurement and performance standards is like setting out on a cross-country trip in a car without a fuel gauge. You can make calculated guesses and assumptions based on experience and observations, but without hard data, conclusions are based on insufficient evidence*"

~ Mikel Harry

Six Sigma Author

The small conference room barely accommodated those in attendance and the heated discussion was making the room feel smaller by the minute. "We already provide exceptional care to our patients. I am not convinced an EMR will change the quality of care we provide," declared a cardiologist. A primary care physician chimed in, "Our margins continue to erode as CMS cuts reimbursement, how can we afford this?" A well respected physician spoke up next, "Productivity may drop as much as 50% after an EMR implementation. What are the plans to compensate us during that time?" These are just a few of the questions on the minds of physicians as they grapple with the changes coming their way.

Physicians spend their days interpreting data from multiple sources and using that information to treat patients. Because they approach problems from an analytical perspective, metrics are one of the most persuasive tools for convincing physicians of the benefits of an EMR accruing directly to their patients and them. In this chapter, we will demonstrate how metrics facilitate physician buy in, improved adoption and meaningful use of an EMR.

· · · Adoption is a prerequisite for · · · meaningful use and we must measure it

According to the HITECH Act legislation, organizations must prove meaningful use of an EMR to earn stimulus monies. The definition of meaningful use continues to evolve, but achieving improved clinical outcomes clearly is the ultimate goal. The details of how it will be administered will surely be debated long into the future. However, despite the ambiguity most are feeling today, it has forced the entire healthcare industry to reconsider how they will implement new technology. As we pointed out in earlier chapters, simply implementing or installing new technology will not be rewarded by stimulus monies – not to mention improved healthcare outcomes.

> "As we pointed out in earlier chapters, simply implementing or installing new technology will not be rewarded by stimulus monies – not to mention improved healthcare outcomes."

Adoption is a prerequisite for meaningful use. A good indicator of a high level of adoption is when everyone is using the EMR according to the organization's prescribed policies and procedures, or best practices. Based on the current legislation, organizations who achieve adoption should be in direct alignment with the intention of meaningful use: improving clinical outcomes.

In Chapter Five, *Using Speed to Proficiency to Create a Training Renaissance*, we discussed a methodology to achieve end user adoption, but following the methodology isn't enough. The only way to know that end users have actually adopted the EMR is to measure their progress. It is clear from our research that very few organizations are measuring adoption. Without measurement, the organization has only subjective assessments of adoption and no way to establish a plan for improvement. We recognize that 100% adoption is unrealistic due to changes in workflow, staff turnover and upgrades, but organizations with the highest rates of adoption will certainly achieve the greatest return on their investment in both clinical and financial terms.

> "The only way to know that end users have actually adopted the EMR is to measure their progress."

The first indicator of adoption is end user proficiency

How would most of us answer the question "Are our end users proficient in the tasks required to use the EMR?" Many organizations assume their training and education will automatically produce end users with a high level of knowledge and confidence in their ability to use new technology, indicating proficiency in their role. But they don't measure the outcomes of their education and training programs. This is a critical step, but one that most organizations don't even consider. Forgoing measurement of end user proficiency means passing on the chance to identify gaps in adoption and ultimately achieve improved clinical and financial

> "Forgoing measurement of end user proficiency means passing on the chance to identify gaps in adoption and ultimately achieve improved clinical and financial outcomes."

outcomes. Proficiency is a key indicator of end user ability to use new technology.

Simulators are an excellent tool for teaching because they not only allow individuals to learn new information in the most effective way, but also provide consistent information to all users. Additionally, they capture valuable data about users' ability to complete role-based tasks in the new system. Data collected by simulators improves education and training programs,

> "Simulators are an excellent tool for teaching because they not only allow individuals to learn new information in the most effective way, but also provide consistent information to all users."

prevents the decay in knowledge commonly experienced after a single training event and ensures EMR access is only granted when a user is proficient in the new application.

We also strongly believe that the combination of high knowledge and confidence produces lasting adoption. The confidence level of employees is highly correlated with long-term adoption. In general, users rate their confidence level as either poor or fair when they are introduced to a new system. As their knowledge increases, their confidence begins to increase. In fact, confidence quickly becomes the driver for achieving higher levels of knowledge. Consider the use of a new technology, like a cell phone. Deciding to upgrade an archaic 2-year old phone to the latest and greatest, feature-rich cell phone quickly causes the realization that the tasks mastered on the old phone function differently on the new phone. Knowledge is low and confidence is in the tank. Watching the demo feature provided on the phone improves knowledge, and soon the new phone's basic functions become easier to master. New-found confidence actually fuels one's willingness to explore new functionality. The interplay between knowledge and confidence is something we all experience daily as we learn.

We recommend collecting baseline data for knowledge and confidence and measuring it again after go-live and at regular intervals thereafter. Our data suggests that organizations should strive for 90-95% of the end users in the excellent or good category for both knowledge and confidence. Once they achieve that milestone, it is time to examine performance metrics in terms of clinical and financial outcomes.

Performance metrics, the clinical and financial outcomes, demonstrate the value of adoption

From a metrics perspective, the most challenging and valuable process is the measurement of what we call performance metrics, valuable because these are the clinical and financial outcomes that drove the organization to purchase an EMR. This is often a daunting task because organizations must customize measurements to represent their specific desired outcomes. Examples of these metrics can include increased adherence to clinical guidelines, increased revenue from improved accuracy in charge capture, reduction in transcription costs and increased RVUs per physician per month. These are among the metrics that will truly validate the investment in an EMR.

Figure 6.1 illustrates the role of performance metrics in the adoption model. Once we have achieved a high level of end user proficiency, the data in the EMR will provide fertile ground for examining the clinical and financial outcomes. The performance metrics will also reinforce the continued effort of keeping leaders engaged and maintaining our process for educating the end users. As we discussed early in this chapter, metrics can also motivate end users to change their behavior. If they are used correctly, a dashboard of relevant and timely metrics will become the focus of the EMR effort.

The first step is to identify the key performance metrics. Most organizations begin the EMR selection process with a formal justification for purchasing their EMR, often in the form of a business case. A strong business case identifies measurable critical outcomes from the EMR. To simplify the process, use research questions to formulate desired outcomes. For example, "Is the EMR reducing personnel, chart supplies and storage costs in the medical records department?"

Once the performance metrics have been identified, the real work begins: capturing the appropriate data. Unfortunately, most EMR vendors do not provide data reports with the level of detail required to track metrics. Designing a methodology for capturing the data required to address the key metrics is complex. The expertise of a trained clinical researcher and often a statistician is very valuable in designing, analyzing and summarizing the data. The commitment to identify even just a few key metrics will provide

Figure 6.1: Adoption Model - Engaged Leadership, Proficient Clinicians & Users, Performance Metrics

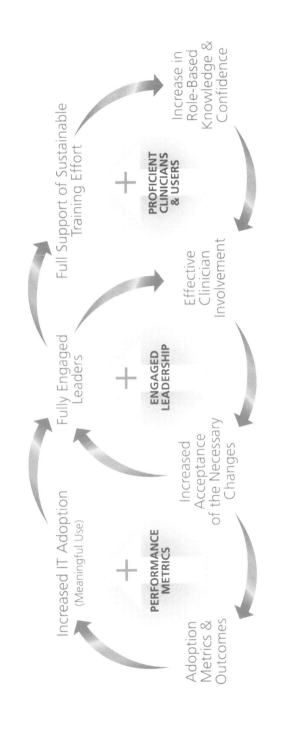

enormous value to the organization. First, it will be very handy in proving meaningful use. Second, it can be used as a dashboard for measuring the performance of the EMR for the life of the application. Most importantly, it will drive continual improvement in the specific areas of value to the organization. It will also create the discipline to assess the value of all health information technology investments objectively.

● ● ● Performance metrics drive the ● ● ● organization to optimize use of the EMR

The meaningful use criteria were born out of a desire to elevate EMR implementations from an IT project to a strategic organizational initiative tied directly to improving healthcare outcomes. It is less about chasing the dollars and more about going the last mile to make a difference in the patient's health! Throughout our country, we can find examples of healthcare organizations at various stages of EMR adoption. Each has the opportunity to improve on key performance metrics. Organizations that measure their performance and maintain the tenacity to continually improve will be rewarded with a stellar reputation, loyal employees and clinical and financial success.

> **"It is less about chasing the dollars and more about going the last mile to make a difference in the patient's health!"**

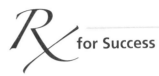

for Success

- Measure employee knowledge and confidence to gauge their level of proficiency.
- Develop a "dashboard" to consistently measure, analyze and communicate key clinical and financial outcomes.
- Commit to utilizing these performance metrics to identify areas of improvement and focus on solutions that actually improve adoption.

95

96

Achieving Lasting Value from IT Adoption

Chapter Preview:
- Most organizations grossly underestimate the effort and resources required to sustain IT adoption.
- Measurements of end user adoption reliably predict improvements and regression in adoption.
- Resources, communications, education and metrics must be shared, updated and easy to find for the life of the application.

" *"The secret of success is constancy of purpose."*

~ Benjamin Disraeli

Several years ago, a reputable IT vendor offered us free use of their software. The software provided monitoring of equipment that would be valuable to us. Initially, we were excited. The functionality aligned with our needs exactly, and the application was robust enough to grow with us. We had a need and the software fulfilled the need. The system served IT directly, so our Director of IT led the implementation and kept our senior management team updated on the progress. We couldn't wait to have access to the dashboard of data promised by the vendor. Months after the implementation, we were still waiting. Although the "free" price tag was alluring, we quickly recognized that the actual maintenance costs and labor required to make the application truly valuable to our organization were lacking. This story drives home a concept that we all understand, but often overlook. Underestimating the "care and feeding" required to maintain a valuable investment puts the entire project at risk. It

> **"Underestimating the 'care and feeding' required to maintain a valuable investment puts the entire project at risk."**

sounds simple, but we all need to remember the importance of sustainability even when initially getting excited about the value of an investment. It is common to under-appreciate the effort it will take to maintain the value of something, even something that initially costs nothing.

Most organizations grossly underestimate the effort and resources required to sustain IT adoption

Let's consider the shift in thinking required to move from implementing an EMR to maintaining high levels of adoption over the life of the application. This is analogous to the shift required to sustain long-term weight maintenance after successful weight loss. The findings from a recent telehealth study are applicable here (Haugen, 2007). The percentage of overweight adults in the U.S. is staggering and continues to rise. Today, over 66 percent of adults in the United States are overweight (Centers for Disease Control, 2006) and 59 percent of Americans are actively trying to lose weight (America On The Move Foundation, 2007). But the problem isn't weight loss! Many of us have successfully lost weight, but can't keep the weight off. As a matter of fact, we regain all the weight (and often more) within 3-5 years (Wadden, 1993; Kramer, 1989). This isn't a complex concept: dieting doesn't incent long-term lifestyle change, thus the weight re-gain. As a result of the initial findings, an innovative program was developed to keep people engaged at various levels depending on their progression through the program. The researchers knew that people needed to practice weight management behaviors actively - for years, not months.

In the world of EMR adoption, we have taken the "dieting" approach to implementing new software solutions in our healthcare settings for too long. We prepared for a go-live event. After go-live, we fell back into our comfortable old habits - resulting in workarounds, regression to ineffective workflows, insufficient training for new users, poor communication and errors. The process of adoption requires a radically different discipline, and the real work begins at go-live. After the successful implementation of a new technology, our tendency is to move on to the next project.

> "The process of adoption requires a radically different discipline, and the real work begins at go-live."

We are busy juggling multiple projects and we actually feel some relief in moving it off our list of highest priorities. A sustainment plan addresses two important areas. First, it establishes how the organization will support the ongoing needs of the end users for the life of the application. This includes communication, education and maintenance of materials and resources. Second, it establishes how and when metrics will be collected to assess end user adoption and performance. Lack of planning and execution in these two areas will lead to a slow and steady deterioration in end user adoption over time.

Effective sustainability plans require resources, time and money. Keep in mind that adoption is never static; it is either improving or degrading in the organization. Figure 7.1 (page 102) illustrates the dynamic nature of adoption over the life cycle of an application. Drops in proficiency appear after upgrades or changes to the application. Leadership must plan for the investment and fund it if their ultimate goal is improved performance. Most organizations only achieve modest adoption after a go-live event, and it takes re-

101

lentless focus to achieve the levels of adoption needed to improve quality of care, patient safety and financial outcomes. Sustainability plans are most successful when they are part of the initial budgeting and planning stages for an EMR.

Figure 7.1: The Life Cycle of Adoption

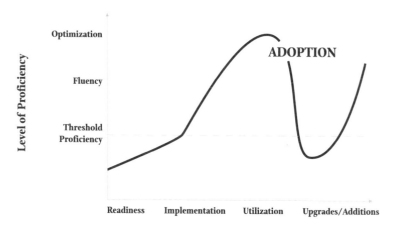

● ● ● Measurements of end user adoption ● ● ● reliably predict improvements and regression in adoption

Sustainment is more than simply maintaining the status quo. If sustainment becomes a passive process of maintenance, it is a waste of resources. Metrics are the differentiating factor between a highly effective sustainment plan and one that is just mediocre. End user knowledge and confidence metrics serve as a barometer for their level of proficiency, providing the earliest indication of adoption, or use of the application according to the organization's best practices. Ultimately, performance metrics are powerful indicators of whether end users are improving, maintaining or regressing in their adoption of the system. If we get an early warning that proficiency is slipping, we can react quickly to address the problem. These metrics are the balancing force for the entire adoption model. As shown in Figure 7.2, this balancing loop, measuring proficiency and performance, ensures that all three of the reinforcing feedback loops continue in a positive direction. Remember, the reinforcing loops are always at risk of moving in the opposite direction and creating barriers or degradation of EMR adoption. Metrics act just as the scale does in long-term weight management; they are the first indicator that we are falling back into old behaviors that are not consistent with sustainable adoption.

> "Ultimately, performance metrics are powerful indicators of whether end users are improving, maintaining or regressing in their adoption of the system."

103

Figure 7.2: Sustainable Solution to EMR Adoption

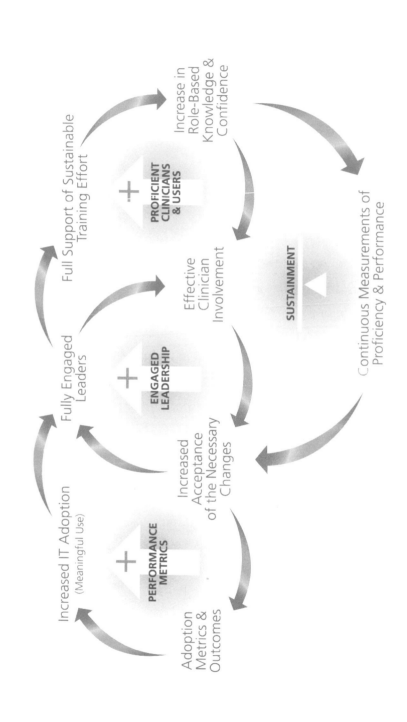

Metrics also keep us on track when performance metrics do not meet expectations. Let's consider two different scenarios to illustrate this idea. In both scenarios, the go-live event was successful, but specific performance metrics do not meet expectations. In most cases, the performance metrics are not achieved because the system is not being utilized effectively. This may be due to inadequate training and therefore lower proficiency, or a problem with the actual performance by end users in the system. Measuring end user proficiency allows us to identify "pockets" of low proficiency among certain users or departments and make sure they receive the education needed. Once users are proficient, we can refocus our attention on the performance metrics. The second scenario is less common, but also more difficult to diagnose. Sometimes users are proficient, but specific performance metrics are still not meeting our expectations. In this case, we need to analyze the specific metric. Are we asking the right question? Are we collecting the right data? Are we examining a very small change or a rare occurrence? There may also be a delay in achieving certain metrics, especially if the measurements are examining small changes. A normal delay can wreak havoc if we start throwing quick fixes at the problem. In this situation, staying the course and having confidence in the metrics will bring desired results.

Resources, communications, education and metrics must be shared, updated and easy to find for the life of the application

Executives, managers and clinicians must continue to lead EMR adoption long after the initial implementation. This is a difficult task because of typical time and resource constraints in healthcare, but achieving the highest levels of adoption will require innovative, efficient and effective solutions to these common problems.

Our research indicates that the ability to achieve and sustain high adoption over time is impacted by turnover, staff growth, workflow changes, application updates and the human factors that impact individual learning and retention. How do we determine the funds and resources needed to overcome these factors? First, consider what the users will need to maintain high levels of knowledge and confidence in using the EMR. Answering a series of questions can be quite effective in helping understand the needs of the users:

- How can we effectively communicate updates and changes in workflow to the users?

> "Executives, managers and clinicians must continue to lead EMR adoption long after the initial implementation. This is a difficult task because of typical time and resource constraints in healthcare, but achieving the highest levels of adoption will require innovative, efficient and effective solutions to these common problems."

- How will we educate new users?
- How will we update quick reference guides or course materials?
- When will metrics be collected and how will they be used?

Second, consider the best approach for meeting these needs. Most organizations are already stretching their resources to the limit, and they assume more resources are required to achieve sustainment. Instead, they should consider how technology can be used to expand their reach in the organization.

Imagine a place dedicated to sustaining EMR adoption in the organization, uncluttered by every update, communication and document from every project; this place would focus solely on improving and sustaining the adoption of an EMR. It would encompass many tools including a learning management system, document management and search capability, communication posts, the ability to plan and archive meetings and much more. Most importantly, it would be incredibly valuable to the end users: easy to access, relevant and meaningful.

> "Imagine a place dedicated to sustaining EMR adoption in the organization, uncluttered by every update, communication and document from every project; this place would focus solely on improving and sustaining the adoption of an EMR."

Based on our work with healthcare clients who struggled with sustainment, we developed a solution that addresses many of the barriers to lasting adoption. We started by identifying the critical tools and resources required to meet the needs of users and then we made it easy to access and use. The concept is a community created to deliver value directly to the end users.

The community is located within a website that looks like a virtual landscape of a unique healthcare organization. Each activity in the community is represented by visible locations in the landscape. For example, the library houses important reference documents and materials. It is easy for a new user to understand that if they want to look something up about a job or task, they simply enter the library and look for the related document (see Figure 7.3). They can read it from their computer screen, print it out, or save it for later use. Each community also includes an auditorium where users can find valuable resources, tools and activities appropriate to the function they currently need, such as videos, virtual meetings and archived events. All online courses or task-based simulators are housed in an education center. The task-based simulators help users become proficient in the tasks they must perform in the system, and they are updated regularly to reflect changes in workflow. The community takes complicated processes and tools and makes them easy to use. This approach offers significant advantages for overcoming the time and resource constraints felt by many organizations around sustainability. It gives the users access to timely, relevant and valuable information. The community eases the strain on resources, but still requires a commitment to the care and feeding of each element if it is going to support lasting end user adoption.

Figure 7.3: PromisePoint Community

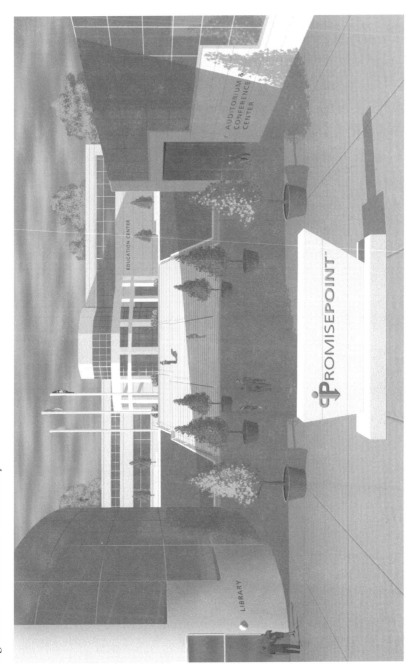

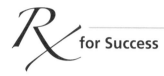

for Success

- Plan now for sustainment by committing appropriate resources, time and funds.
- Develop a reporting and analysis process to determine where to focus sustainment efforts.
- Find an innovative solution to expand the reach to end users. A web-based community is an example of a technology that gives users timely, relevant and valuable information.

110

CHAPTER EIGHT

The Journey Continues...

112

Now that we have presented a methodology for lasting adoption, let us return to the story of UT Medical Group to demonstrate some of these ideas in practice.

We are now in the midst of our second implementation or "re-implementation" as we refer to it. My highest priority before beginning the re-implementation was to recruit a new Chief Information Officer (CIO). I decided that only candidates who had experience in managing or implementing an EMR, preferably in an ambulatory setting, should be considered. Further, I decided that our IT staff and medical leaders would be actively involved, to a degree greater than ordinarily expected, throughout the recruiting process. It was critical that the candidates meet the team up front and understand our position. I wanted to make absolutely certain that the new CIO was completely open to the challenge of leading a re-implementation. We were very lucky to have had several excellent candidates from which to choose. Once we found the right person, our journey to adoption continued.

I am optimistic, if not ecstatic, about where we are today and with what we have accomplished, in part thanks to one very big change between the initial implementation and our "re-implementation". We established a formal governance structure specific to the EMR project that includes all stakeholders. There is a Steering Committee, a Physicians Advisory Group (PAG), a Nursing Advisory Committee and a Touch-Works Leaders Group. The overall project responsibility resides in the Steering Committee, comprised of the organization's executive officers and the chairs of the PAG, the Nursing Advisory Committee and the TouchWorks Leaders Group. The TouchWorks Leaders Group includes leaders from clinics, compliance, medical records, privacy, marketing, credentialing and enrollment and IT.

The PAG has a wide range of physicians, including some who initially opposed the EMR. At least one doctor represents each department, with larger departments having two representatives. The Dean of the College of Medicine and Chairman of the Board for UTMG empowered the PAG to be the sole developer and communicator for all policies related to the EMR at UTMG. A major reason I believe we are successful today is that the Dean consistently reinforced the message that the use of the EMR was not optional; everyone would use it according to the established policies. We intentionally decided that neither the Board nor the CEO should make policies around how to use the system as physician leadership and ownership was deemed a critical success factor. Although working through issues is painful at times, the PAG continues in its leadership role with respect to development and implementation for policy decisions to ensure that each policy has been fully considered by those who are most familiar with the EMR, and those who will ultimately use the EMR.

Additionally, there was a level of prestige accorded to those who were part of the PAG. Physician leadership and governance has been incredibly important to our success, and once this group understood and embraced its charter, the re-implementation really began to take off. People want the system to work and for it to work well. Some even made a competition out of how fast everyone in the department

> "Physician leadership and governance has been incredibly important to our success, and once this group understood and embraced its charter, the re-implementation really began to take off. "

could adopt. There were no more questions about if we would adopt; we all were on the same page of getting it done. And we have done so with reasonable success; the medical staff ownership in the EMR is growing, while administration and IT provide support as needed. We look forward to the day when the medical staff promotes the use of the EMR and considers it an absolute necessary element of providing quality care.

During the first implementation, UTMG did not have the PAG to provide direction to our departments and programs. Some wanted all their records scanned in, some did not and everyone proceeded with what they thought best for their department. Inconsistency was the rule of the day. Today there are policies in place for the use of the EMR, including which records to scan, standard screen alerts and appropriate levels of customization within departments. The PAG also established the policy that requires physicians to show proficiency in use of the EMR through their training; if they do not, they are denied access to the EMR. There is even an escalation policy involving the department chair and CMO that can result in disciplinary action, if necessary, until training is completed. The PAG has also established policies of EMR use by residents and medical students. Our communications have improved as well. We ensure that all policy notices regarding physician use of the EMR come directly from the PAG, rather than from IT, so that departments understand that the PAG really governs this initiative and that we are all aligned.

Another significant difference in our approach was in the training methodology. In our initial effort, we worked with a training vendor who used a standard lecture series with a traditional train-the-trainer method. There were a number of reasons that this method was not effective for our organization and in our environment. Users did not retain the information, and the information taught was not always consistent. Physicians and staff spent hours away from patient care responsibilities to attend training and often still were not able to perform their role-specific tasks in the system once they returned to work. We knew there must be a more effective training methodology.

In the re-implementation, we were fortunate enough to begin with a new vision for helping healthcare providers spend less time learning technology and more time treating patients. The Breakaway Group assisted us with engaging our leaders, establishing a communication plan, developing role- and task-specific online learning, using metrics to track adoption and providing a plan for sustainability. The interactive learning system allowed us to certify that users demonstrated the required proficiency level before being permitted to use the new system. In addition, our IT team developed and provided a production environment for users to practice tasks according to prescribed workflows. This complements the online learning tools.

We had not appreciated the differences in training required by different roles. We now employ online task-based simulators for each major role in our organization. It made so much sense; why require someone to take a course not needed for their job? The wonderful thing about online accessibility is that it allowed anyone to train anywhere, any time. It also allowed UTMG to track individual proficiency and completion of training. As we progress, I am also seeing new staff adopting the system quite easily, never falling into the old way of

> "As we progress, I am also seeing new staff adopting the system quite easily, never falling into the old way of paper charting."

paper charting. With online learning, new employees simply complete the assigned learning, ensuring that they are up to speed on our EMR. The combination of online availability and specificity of training provided a superior method of getting staff up to speed.

We also believe super users play an important role. Our CIO and IT team developed a program where we train select physicians and clinic staff in all functions of the system rather than those few that pertain to their role. They then provide at-the-elbow assistance in the clinics. We have had great success with this program; super users receive recognition for their extra effort, and we know that all users receive full support.

Lastly, we better understand the importance of metrics in evaluating end user adoption across the organization. Most of us agree that it is difficult to manage what is not measured. So it is here. Monitoring EMR use or lack thereof is critical. It allows us to track progress toward the goals established for our organization, clinicians and patients. Some of our metrics include our ability to decrease dictation and transcription costs over time, the number of electronic versus paper prescriptions written, and the number of users actively employing order entry, to name a few. Our metrics are designed to monitor improvements in quality of care and organizational efficiency.

> "Lastly, we better understand the importance of metrics in evaluating end user adoption across the organization. Most of us agree that it is difficult to manage what is not measured."

It is noteworthy that this experience offered important lessons regarding how to best prepare for future projects at UTMG. We learned how to focus the entire organization's attention on one objective. It was our first experience with a major league culture and leadership change project with all the elements: engaged leadership, clear governance, a charter and accountabilities. Today we understand that engaging leaders must include establishing and reaching agreement on the overall objective, communicating regularly and consistently on a broad basis and conducting the implementation in a fair and equitable manner.

> "Today we understand that engaging leaders must include establishing and reaching agreement on the overall objective, communicating regularly and consistently on a broad basis and conducting the implementation in a fair and equitable manner."

The most important lessons learned through this long process now seem intuitive. Technology implementation and adoption is a project of equal parts culture change, communication and technology. To that end, I intellectually knew but underappreciated the following:

1) When the Board and the medical leadership in our organization united in communicating a positive message about the change, it had a critical impact. Together we insisted that everyone embrace the new technology, that we recognized it would be difficult, but that we were going to do it nonetheless.

2) Having structured governance in place with a Physicians Advisory Group made it possible to set defined and consistent expectations across the organization and

provided leadership and constructive criticism critical to project success.

3) Although challenging at times, everyone must remain focused on the goal and committed to the outcome. In order to succeed, defensiveness and finger pointing can't be tolerated.

4) When IT is the driving force behind an EMR implementation, the organization contributes to a doomed project. We needed the entire organization to make the commitment, and to get to that point, we needed to involve everyone, especially the clinicians. The communication plan was vital to our success.

While I like to think we have it all figured out now, the acquisition, implementation and adoption of any new technology is a journey of many steps. We know that all new staff will learn how to use our EMR consistently and according to uniform policies. The time it will take for them to get up to speed is much shorter, allowing them to spend more time treating patients and less time on the computer. I am thrilled to say that we have truly improved our organization and its operation to the ultimate benefit of our patients.

--Steven Burkett, UT Medical Group

The story of UT Medical Group is compelling not only because it demonstrates the real-life challenges of EMR adoption, but more importantly because it shows how focusing on adoption can dramatically improve the outcomes. It also reminds us that adoption is not a destination; we must relentlessly pursue adoption over the life of the application. UT Medical Group is fully aware of the work that still needs to be done to achieve their long-term goals and maintain a high level of adoption.

The methodology for achieving adoption begins with engaged leaders; their charge is to establish a new leadership agenda focused on EMR adoption. Their efforts will establish the necessity of educating the end users and ensuring their proficiency in the EMR. Once all end users achieve a high level of proficiency, it is much easier to establish, track and utilize performance metrics. As the clinical and financial outcomes begin to show the intended benefits from the EMR, we can optimize and manage the use of the EMR. Those metrics are also critical indicators of our ability to sustain adoption long-term. As we build momentum within each component of the model, our efforts are rewarded by increased engagement, improved proficiency among end users and ultimately a higher quality of care.

The prescription for lasting adoption isn't a pill, it is a regimen that requires discipline and hard work, but it will result in the lasting adoption of an EMR.

> **"The prescription for lasting adoption isn't a pill, it is a regimen that requires discipline and hard work, but it will result in the lasting adoption of an EMR."**

Aldrich, C. (2000). The Justification of IT Training. Gartner Research Note DF-11-3614. Retrieved from http://clarkaldrich.blogspot.com/ 2007/01/clark-aldrich-bio.html

Amarasingham, R., Plantinga, L., Diener-West, M., Gaskin, D., Powe, N. (2009, January 26). Clinical information technologies and inpatient outcomes: a multiple hospital study. *Archives of Internal Medicine*, 169(2):108-114.

America on the Move Foundation (AOMF). (2007, September). New Research From America On the Move Foundation Indicates American Weight Loss Efforts Stalling. Retrieved from http://www.prnewswire. com/cgi-bin/stories.pl?ACCT=109&STORY=/www/story/09-12-2007/0004661618&EDATE=.

American College of Physicians (ACP). (2008). Medicare 2008 Pay-for-Reporting Program. Retrieved from http://www.acponline.org/ running_practice/practice_management/payment_coding/pqri_ desc_07.pdf.

American Medical Informatics Assocation (AMIA). (2006, June 13). A Roadmap for National Action on Clinical Decision Support. Retrieved from http://www.amia.org/inside/initiatives/cds.

American Society for Training and Development (ASTD). (2009). Annual Survey. Retrieved from http://maamodt.asp.radford.edu/HR%20Statistics/dollars_spent_on_training.htm

Asbjörnson, K. (2008, January). Conversation with Charles Fred on Exploring Inspired Leadership Through Music. http://www.inspirei-magineinnovate.com/Inspiring-Performance.asp

Asch, S., McGlynn, E., Hogan, M., Hayward, R., Shekelle, P., et al. (2004, December 21). Comparison of Quality of Care for Patients in the Veterans Health Administration and Patients in a National Sample. *Annals of Internal Medicine*, 141(12):938-945.

Audet, A., Doty, M., Peugh, J., Shamasdin, J., Zapert, K., et al. (2004). Information technologies: when will they make it into physicians' black bags? *Medscape General Medicine*, 6(4):2.

Burleson, D. (2001, August 16). Four Factors that Shape the Cost of ERP. Retrieved from http://www.dba-oracle.com/art_erp_factors.htm

Centers for Disease Control (CDC), National Center for Health Statistics (NCHS). (2006, April). Prevalence of Overweight and Obesity Among Adults: United States, 2003-2004. Retrieved from http://www.cdc.gov/nchs/products/pubs/pubd/hestats/overweight/overwght_adult_03.htm

Centers for Medicare and Medicaid Services (CMS), U.S. Department of Health & Human Services (HHS). (2009, November 18). Electronic Prescribing (eRx) Incentive Program. Retrieved from http://www.cms.hhs.gov/ERxIncentive/.

Centers for Medicare and Medicaid Services (CMS), U.S. Department of Health & Human Services (HHS). (2009, January). What's New for the 2009 Physician Quality Reporting Initiative (PQRI). Retrieved from http://www.cms.hhs.gov/PQRI/Downloads/PQRIWhatsNew2009Final.pdf.

Chen, C., Garrido, T., Chock, D., Okawa, G., Liang, L. (2009). The Kaiser Permanente Electronic Health Record: Transforming and Streamlining Modalities of Care. Health Affairs, 28(2), 323-333.

Congress of the United States, Congressional Budget Office (CBO). (2008, May). Evidence on the Costs and Benefits of Health Information Technology: A CBO Paper.

CoverMD. (2009). Electronic Medical Records: A Way to Save Money on Your Malpractice Insurance. Retrieved from www.covermd.com/resources/electronic-medical-records-medmal-insurance.aspx

DesRoches, C., Campbell, E., Rao, S., Donelan, K., Ferris, T., et al. (2008, July 3). Electronic health records in ambulatory care--a national survey of physicians. *New England Journal of Medicine*, 359(1), 50-60. Retrieved from http://www.ncbi.nlm.nih.gov/pubmed/18565855?ordinalpos=1&itool=EntrezSystem2.PEntrez.Pubmed.Pubmed_ResultsPanel.Pubmed_DefaultReportPanel.Pubmed_RVDocSum

Florida Medical Quality Assurance, Inc. (FMQAI). (2008). Physician Practice Resource Manual: Doctor's Office Quality – Information Technology – 8th Scope of Work, August 1, 2005-July 31, 2008.

Fred, C. (2002). Breakaway. Jossey-Bass: San Francisco.

Gillette, B. (2006, March 1). Industrywide EMR adoption accelerates as barriers are overcome. *Managed Healthcare Executive for Decision Makers in Healthcare*. Retrieved from http://license.icopyright.net/user/viewFreeUse.act?fuid=Mzc1OTQ0Mg%3D%3D

Gladwell, M. (2002). *The Tipping Point: How Little Things Can Make a Big Difference.* Little Brown and Company: New York.

Grieger, D., Cohen, S., Krusch, D. (2007, February 28). A Pilot Study to Document the Return on Investment for Implementing an Ambulatory Electronic Health Record at an Academic Medical Center. *Journal of the American College of Surgeons*, 205(1), 89-96. doi:10.1016/j.jamcollsurg.2007.02.074

Haugen, H., Tran, Z., Wyatt, H., Barry, M., Hill, J. (2007, December). Using Telehealth to Increase Participation in Weight Maintenance Programs. Obesity 15(12), 3067–3077. doi: 10.1038/oby.2007.365

Institute of Medicine (IOM). (1999, November). To Err is Human: Building a Safer Health System. Retrieved from http://www.nap.edu/books/0309068371/html/

James, R. (2009, June 10). Jim Collins: How Mighty Companies Fall. *TIME Magazine*. Retrieved from http://www.time.com/time/business/article/0,8599,1903713,00.html

Jha, A., Ferris, T., Donelan, K., DesRoches, C., Shields, A., et al. (2006, October 11). How common are electronic health records in the United States? A summary of the evidence. *Health Affairs*, 25(6), w496-507. Retrieved from http://www.ncbi.nlm.nih.gov/pubmed/17035341?ordinalpos=39&itool=EntrezSystem2.PEntrez.Pubmed.Pubmed_ResultsPanel.Pubmed_DefaultReportPanel.Pubmed_RVDocSum. doi: 10.1377/hlthaff.25.w496

Kolb, David A. (1984). *Experiential Learning*. Prentice Hall: New Jersey.

Kramer, F., Jeffery, R., Forster, J., Snell, M. (1989). Long-term follow-up of behavioral treatment for obesity: patterns of weight regain among men and women. *International Journal of Obesity and Related Metabolic Disorders*, 13, 123-136.

Massachusetts Technology Cooperative, New England Healthcare Institute (NEHI). (2008). Saving Lives, Saving Money: the imperative for computerized physician order entry in Massachusetts hospitals. Retrieved from http://www.nehi.net/publications/8/saving_lives_saving_money_the_imperative_for_computerized_physician_order_entry_in_massachusetts_hospitals

McGlynn, E., Asch, S., Adams, J., Keesey, J., Hicks, J., et al. (2003, June 26). The Quality of Health Care Delivered to Adults in the United States. *New England Journal of Medicine*, 348, 2635-2645.

Medical Informatics Engineering. (2010). Medical Informatics Engineering today announced the addition of a Physician Quality Reporting Initiative (PQRI) module to its WebChart electronic medical record system. Retrieved from http://www.mieweb.com/news/posts/78 ?searched=pqri+module&advsearch=oneword&highlight=ajaxSear ch_highlight+ajaxSearch_highlight1+ajaxSearch_highlight2

Miller, R., Sim, I. (2004, March/April). Physicians' Use of Electronic Medical Records: Barriers and Solutions. *Health Affairs*, 23(2), 116-126. doi: 10.1377/hlthaff.23.2.116

Miller, R., West, C., Brown, T., Sim, I., Ganchoff, C. (2005, September/October). The value of electronic health records in solo or small group practices. *Health Affairs*, 24(5), 112-137. doi: 10.1377/hlthaff.24.5.1127

National Coalition on Health Care (NCHC). (2009, July 17). Health Insurance Costs. Retrieved from http://www.nchc.org/facts/cost.shtml

Nationwide Health Information Network (NHIN). (2009, July 17). Over view. Retrieved from http://healthit.hhs.gov/portal/server.pt?open= 512&objID=1142&parentname=CommunityPage&parentid=2&mode =2&in_hi_userid=10741&cached=true

Organisation for Economic Co-operation and Development (OECD) Health Division. (2008). OECD Health Data, December, 2008.

Parapundit.com. (2006, June 25). Physician incomes declining while people use them more. Retrieved from http://www.parapundit.com/archives/003541.html

Senge, P. (1994). *The Fifth Discipline*. Doubleday: New York.

THINKMAP Visual Thesaurus. (2010). Retrieved from http://www. visualthesaurus.com/

Tu, H., Ginsburg, P. (2006, June). Losing Ground: Physician Income, 1995- 2003. Center for Studying Health System Change: Tracking Report No. 15. Retrieved from http://hschange.com/CONTENT/851/

Virapongse, A., Bates, D., Shi, P., Jenter, C., Volk, L., et al. (2008, November 24). Electronic health records and malpractice claims in office practice. Archives of Internal Medicine, 168(21), 2362-2367.

Wadden, T. (1993). Treatment of obesity by moderate and severe caloric restriction: Results of clinical research trials. *Annals of Internal Medicine*, 119, 688-693.

Wang, S., Middleton, B., Prosser, L., Bardon, C. Spurr, C., et al. (2003, April 1). A Cost-Benefit Analysis of Electronic Medical Records in Primary Care. *The American Journal of Medicine*, 114, 397-403. doi: 10.1016/S0002-9343(03)00057-3

Wheatley, M. (2000, June 1). ERP Training Stinks. *CIO Magazine*. Retrieved from http://www.cio.com/article/148900/ERP_Training_Stinks

Wicklund, E. (2009, March 3). GE Healthcare helps CoxHealth tap into PQRI program. Healthcare IT News. Retrieved from http://www. healthcareitnews.com/news/ge-healthcare-helps-coxhealth-tap-pqri-program

Woolhandler, S., Campbell, T., Himmelstein, D. (2003, August 21). Costs of Health Care Administration in the United States and Canada. *New England Journal of Medicine*, 349(8), 768-775.

LITERATURE REVIEW

Adopting an EMR will improve the organization's quality of care, patient safety and efficiency

We have the opportunity to transform healthcare by providing access to comprehensive medical information that is secure, standardized and shared. A growing body of literature confirms the value of electronic health records (EHRs) in improving patient safety, improving coordination of care, enhancing documentation, reducing administrative inefficiencies, facilitating clinical decision-making and adherence to evidence-based clinical guidelines (Chen et al, 2009; Massachusetts Technology Cooperative, 2008; Amarasingham et al, 2009). This literature review provides some strong evidence for improved clinical and financial outcomes.

Improved quality of care and patient safety

Improved quality of care and patient safety is often the primary driver for EMR adoption. Clinicians strive to provide the highest quality of care and to be vigilant in ensuring the safety of our patients. Yet the IOM Report To Err is Human reports that as many as 98,000 people die each year from medical errors, a staggering statistic to comprehend (Institute of Medicine, 1999). In commercial aviation, this would be the equivalent of one medium-sized airliner crashing every day. Despite our commitment to patient

129

safety, because we are human and because healthcare is extraordinarily complex, taking advantage of improvements in error rates associated with EMR adoption is not something we can afford to pass by.

There is much healthcare can learn from the aviation industry. The Federal Aviation Administration (FAA) mandated Crew Resource Management (CRM) training in 1992. This human factors training focuses on error prevention, recognition and management through teamwork, communication and procedural protocols, and has been a major contributor to a dramatic reduction in commercial aviation accidents.

An EMR can provide analogous benefits to a medical practice. It can contribute to patient safety and quality care by preventing errors (drug-drug interactions), recognizing and helping providers manage errors by alerting them to potential complications of treatment (drug allergies) and providing electronic procedural protocols by flagging abnormal laboratory results and reminding providers to schedule preventative health screenings.

"The quality of health care could be improved through the use of Clinical Decision Support (CDS) systems to remind physicians to schedule tests, help diagnose complicated conditions, and more effectively implement appropriate protocols for treatment (Congressional Budget Office, 2008)."

A recent study examined the effects an EMR can have on patient safety in a primary care setting. An expert panel performed an analysis to determine the potential benefits associated with encounters at an ambulatory medical center. As a result of basic medication decision support, adverse drug events would be reduced by approximately 34 percent (Wang et al, 2003). In a study of 52 family practice offices, the most common errors were in medication selection and dosage. The study concluded that 57% of errors could be prevented. The quality of care received by patients in the VA system, which uses an EHR that includes CDS tools, was superior to that received by a nationally representative sample of the population (Asch et al, 2004). Today doctors often do not have access to the right information at the right time, potentially compromising patient care. EMRs provide instant access to this information 24 hours a day, via any Internet connection.

Enhanced documentation

Accurate charge capture is critical to the financial success of a practice. To avoid allegations of over-coding in an audit, many physicians tend to "under code". Physicians may also fail to document all services adequately, unintentionally under-coding. EMR use promotes more complete documentation and thus more complete capture of services and more defensible coding at higher coding levels (Miller et al, 2004). Documentation legibility is clearly enhanced in an EMR. Other users of the record no longer have to decipher physicians' notoriously poor handwriting, which often results in misinterpretations and errors. Since the medical record is also a legal document, accurate and legible EMR documentation will serve the profession well in legal proceedings.

Cost Savings and Improved Operational Efficiency

Today, about 30 percent of US healthcare dollars go to healthcare administrative costs (Woolhandler et al, 2003). We have an opportunity to decrease the cost of healthcare dramatically simply by reducing operational inefficiencies.

An ambulatory EMR has the potential to be a powerful tool for cost savings and revenue enhancement. Transcription expenses, decreased time and costs expended in telephone calls and facsimile communications and decreased charge filing costs can all be significantly reduced (Gillette, 2006). The opportunity for greatest cost savings in most practices is in medical record management: decreased staffing requirements for chart pulling, filing and maintenance, elimination of cost to build new patient charts and decreased or eliminated chart storage (Audet et al, 2004). Additionally, some evidence exists that physicians using EMRs are less likely to have paid malpractice claims (Virapongse et al, 2008), and many insurers offer premium credits between 2 and 5 percent for EMR users (CoverMD, 2009). Improved operational efficiencies can increase revenue through more accurate coding, more complete capture of provided services and more timely collection of payments (Audet et al, 2004).

The combination of cost savings and increased revenue provide a positive return on investment for an EMR. Primary care practices achieve the breakeven point for recovery of initial and ongoing cumulative costs in 2.5 years, with an ongoing annual "profit" of $23,000 per physician (Miller, 2005). Another study of primary care practices reports a cumulative net benefit of $86,400 per physician over the first five years after EMR implementation (Wang et al, 2003). Similar results have been published for the ambulatory clinics at the University of Rochester Medical Center, with breakeven in 16 months and subsequent annual savings of $10,000 per physician (Grieger et al, 2007).

Facilitating CDS and Adherence to Evidence-Based Clinical Guidelines

Unexplained geographic variations in utilization and cost of local medical care have contributed to the development of evidence-based clinical guidelines (McGlynn et al, 2003). Just keeping abreast of the explosion of new research and treatments is a daunting task, not to mention putting them into practice. It is literally impossible for the human brain to assimilate and apply this continually burgeoning amount of new medical information. Physicians are now turning to technology to provide patient-specific, timely, accurate and current medical knowledge to enhance care. A robust CDS module in an EMR encompasses a variety of tools and interventions, such as computerized alerts, reminders, clinical guidelines, order sets, patient reports and dashboards, documentation templates, diagnostic support and clinical workflow tools (American Medical Informatics Association, 2006). CDS is often the last component of an EMR to be adopted because of the complexity, time investment, effort to gain organizational consensus and clinician resistance to "cookbook medicine"; however, most physicians do recognize the value of timely, accurate and easy to access clinical knowledge.

How the organization chooses to customize and maintain the

module will enhance or degrade its functionality. Excessive or inappropriate alerts and reminders can impede adoption. CDS brings tremendous potential value to organizations committed to fine-tuning the application. Like all technology, the content put in dictates the quality of the result.

Pay for Performance/Physician Quality Reporting Initiative (PQRI)

Medicare's Physician Quality Reporting Initiative (PQRI) for 2009 pays physicians a 2 percent bonus on top of their total allowed charges if they successfully report on at least three quality measures from a designated list of 153 (Centers for Medicare and Medicaid Services, 2009). Adoption of electronic health records is one of these quality measures and physicians that use EHR systems on a regular basis qualify for one of three required measures (American College of Physicians, 2008). There is also a subset of PQRI measures accepted to test the EHR submission process. There is currently no incentive payment associated with this measure; clearly, Medicare's goal is to encourage adoption of EHR reporting for this program (Centers for Medicare and Medicaid Services, 2009). When evaluating EMR vendors, one requirement should be an application that automatically generates the data required for the PQRI voluntary reporting, making qualifying for the 2% bonus payment much easier (Medical Informatics Engineering, 2010; Healthcare IT News, 2009).

Another opportunity to increase the Medicare reimbursement is the 2009 Medicare E-Prescribing Incentive Program. This program is completely separate from PQRI, and it is possible to participate in both. It provides a 2% incentive for using e-prescribing with at least 50% of Medicare cases. Currently, this incentive allows collection of 2% of all Medicare allowable charges, not just those associated with patients for whom e-prescribing was used. E-prescribing is a component of all certified EMRs (Centers for Medicare and Medicaid Services, 2009).

A healthy dose of skepticism will serve us well as we review the EMR literature. Not because it is misleading, but because it doesn't tell the whole story. Considering the strong evidence for EMRs, why haven't more organizations implemented them? Only 17% of physician practices report use of an EMR (DesRoches et al, 2008). Why did we begin this book with a story of poor adoption and outcomes? Why do we continue to hear stories of user resistance, software that isn't ready for prime time, workflow struggles, higher than expected costs and lower than expected revenues, increases in staffing and worse quality metrics? The disconnect between the evidence in the literature and our real-world experiences is borne in the assumption that implementing an EMR and adopting an EMR are synonymous.

Visit ***www.beyondimplementation.org*** for free book excerpts, upcoming events, and more.

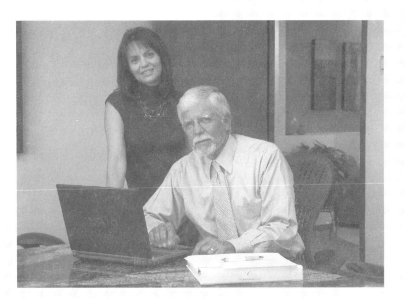

137

Heather A. Haugen, Ph.D, RD   Jeffrey R. Woodside, M.D.

The authors have extensive experience conducting research in the clinical healthcare environment. Their passion and commitment for helping organizations adopt EMRs successfully has guided them through their endeavors to understand how leaders navigate EMR adoption, and led to the findings presented in this book. They have witnessed the outcomes of poor adoption and are committed to helping organizations successfully adopt an EMR, ultimately making healthcare safer and more efficient.

Dr. Heather Haugen has more than fifteen years of research experience in both the academic and private sectors. She earned her doctorate in health information technology from the University of Colorado Health Sciences Center. She has an extensive and diverse professional history that includes grant writing, designing and coordinating clinical trials, research presentations and education and training for numerous healthcare providers.

Haugen's research experience ranges from weight management and metabolism to telehealth and behavior change. She is widely published in health and medical journals, including the Journal of American Dietetic Association, Journal of the American College of Nutrition and International Journal of Obesity. Haugen holds a faculty position with the University of Colorado Health Sciences Center's School of Medicine as the associate track director of health information technology, where she actively conducts research, mentors students and teaches courses.

Haugen is a native of Denver where she lives with her husband and daughter. She enjoys running, hiking and spending time with her family in the beautiful Rocky Mountains.

Dr. Jeffrey R. Woodside is the former executive vice president and chief medical officer for UT Medical Group, Inc. He received his undergraduate degree from Oregon State University and earned his medical degree from the University of Oregon Medical School, where he later interned. Following a stint as a flight surgeon in the U.S. Navy, he completed residencies in general surgery and urology at the University of New Mexico School of Medicine. He also received an M.B.A. from the University of Phoenix.

His career spans more than 30 years and includes faculty appointments at the University of New Mexico School of Medicine in Albuquerque and the University of Texas Medical School in Houston, where he also served as vice president of The Hermann Hospital. In 1992, Woodside was named UT Medical Group's medical director, a position he held until 1995. He was also appointed medical director of UT Bowld Hospital and professor of urology at the University of Tennessee College of Medicine. In 1993, he was named executive director of the UT Medical Center. He was appointed executive vice President and chief medical officer for UTMG and associate dean for clinical affairs for the College of Medicine in 1999.

Woodside has been active in many medical organizations and served as a reviewer for various urology journals. He also served on the Editorial Board for the journal, Neurourology and Urodynamics.

After recently retiring from academic medicine, Woodside and his wife moved to Pickwick Lake, Tennessee. They enjoy community involvement, golfing, fishing, cooking and entertaining family and friends.

139

◆

About Steven H. Burkett

Steven H. Burkett has served as the president and CEO of UTMG and its predecessor organization since early 1984. In that time, he has proven to be a well-respected professional and a visionary leader. A native Arkansan, Burkett has a broad background in academic medical practice and administration, including over 30 years' affiliation with UT Medical Group and the University of Tennessee. For the past 20 years, Burkett has served as adjunct instructor for the Graduate Program in Health Services Administration at the University of Memphis. His publications include Practice Management Courses for Residents: A Contribution to Education and Microcomputer Applications in Academic Medicine. Burkett makes frequent presentations to healthcare associations and other professional organizations regarding various aspects of the healthcare industry. He also served as chairman of the board for Memphis Managed Care Corporation, a TennCare health maintenance organization based in Memphis. Burkett is a member of the Association of American Medical Colleges Group on Faculty Practice, having previously served as Chairperson. He is also an active member of the Medical Group Management Association and the American Group Management Association. Burkett is a founding Board member of the Mid South eHealth Alliance, a regional health information organization based in Memphis, and currently serves as Board Chair.

PRINTED IN THE UNITED STATES

9 780984 205103